THE SECRET OF THE FIVE RITES

THE SECRET OF THE FIVE RITES

In Search of a Lost Western Tradition of Inner Alchemy

John Michael Greer

AEON

First published in 2023 by
Aeon Books

Copyright © 2023 by John Michael Greer

British Library Cataloguing in Publication Data

A C.I.P. for this book is available from the British Library

ISBN-13: 978-1-80152-065-2

Typeset by vPrompt eServices Pvt Ltd, India

www.aeonbooks.co.uk

CONTENTS

INTRODUCTION

In 1939, the Mid-Day Press, a small publishing firm in Los Angeles, issued a thirty-two-page booklet by Peter Kelder titled *The Eye of Revelation*. It taught a simple but effective set of five exercises for health and longevity, the Five Rites. The author claimed that he had learned these from an Englishman he called by the pseudonym of Colonel Bradford, who studied them while staying in a lamasery somewhere in southern Asia, and who had been rejuvenated to a dramatic degree by practicing them.

Certain dietary rules and lifestyle principles accompanied the Rites, so did a Sixth Rite that worked the diaphragm muscles and redirected sexual energies, and so did a set of teachings about seven energy centers or vortices in the body, which are not the same as the well-known seven chakras along the spine. These vortices are among the most distinctive things about the system and are found in only a scattered handful of sources elsewhere. It is by awakening the vortices to their normal rate of spin, the book claims, that the Rites achieve their effects.

Kelder's central claim was that daily practice of the Five Rites would restore health and vigor to the old and maintain these things in the young. He also hinted that the Rites formed the foundation for a set of practices that could open the way to supernormal states of awareness, by means of the redirection of the sexual energies just mentioned. The pamphlet made only brief references to these deeper dimensions, however, and focused primarily on rejuvenation.

The Eye of Revelation was one of many publications on exercise and spirituality that saw print that year. Plenty of those other books first saw print in California, too. By the time Kelder's booklet was published, the Golden State had been a hotbed of alternative culture and esoteric spirituality for more than two decades. Health food stores and occult-themed bookstores in California and elsewhere put the booklet on the shelves alongside competing volumes. At the time, it apparently didn't sell enough copies to merit a second printing.

In 1946, the Mid-Day Press issued an expanded edition with two further chapters. This had no more of an impact on the world than the original edition. Today both editions are rarities: only two copies of the 1939 edition and only one copy of the 1946 edition are known to exist. In the bustling and highly competitive world of American alternative spirituality, they were apparently one more flash in the pan.

That began to change in 1975 when Borderland Sciences Research Foundation—a California-based network of researchers interested in the places where science and spirituality overlap—issued an inexpensive reprint of the 1939 edition. Thereafter the Five Rites began to show up in other publications, notably Donald Michael Kraig's bestselling 1985 occult textbook *Modern Magick*. By the turn of the millennium, as interest in the exercises spread, the Rites were being practiced by individuals and taught by exercise teachers all over the world. Since then the same process has only accelerated.

All this interest inevitably stirred up questions about the origins of the Five Rites and the teachings that framed them. The book's claim that the Rites originated in a lamasery somewhere near India sparked many attempts to trace the origins of the exercises to a Tibetan source, without any noticeable success. Various other theories were floated without ever settling the matter, and in the usual way of things, the controversies stirred up tempests in an assortment of online teapots. One difficulty that none of these theories were able to cope with was the simple fact that the Five Rites do not appear to have been taught anywhere in the Indian subcontinent or the Himalayan regions before Kelder published his book.

All the theories of the Five Rites' origins, as far as I know, looked east to the healing arts and mystical traditions of Asia. All the while, the solution to the riddle was waiting unnoticed in a very different place.

The Western world has its own healing arts and mystical traditions, its own systems of energy centers and exercises for awakening them, but it has also a very complex and conflicted relationship with these arts, traditions, and systems. It therefore became fashionable in the nineteenth and twentieth centuries to claim Eastern origins for Western traditions. Since it was equally fashionable during these same years for Western mystics and occultists to draw on Eastern sources when they could, a great deal of confusion inevitably resulted. The origins of the Five Rites were among the things that got caught up in that confusion. Despite the story Peter Kelder told in *The Eye of Revelation*, the Rites originated in the West, not in the East; they drew some of their inspiration from material about Indian spiritual practices available in the American occult community in the 1930s, but they are a Western creation, and more specifically an American creation.

It needs to be remembered that today's sensitivities about cultural appropriation did not yet exist in 1939. At that time, and for decades before and after, references to Asian countries were used constantly to add the exotic cachet of distant lands to homegrown American products. Stores that carried "spiritual supplies" in the African-American neighborhoods of greater Los Angeles in the year *The Eye of Revelation* was first published, for example, sold bottles of Hindu Grass Oil and Chinese Wash—two widely used ingredients in urban folk magic that had no connection to India or China except the names.

In that same year, visitors to Laguna Beach could take in lectures from an occult society called the Royal Order of Tibet, which had no more to do with Tibet than it did with royalty. (Its head was George Adamski, who would become much more famous a decade later as the most successful of the first generation of UFO contactees.) The lamasery that played a central role in the origin story of the Five Rites, as we will see, was one more example of the same custom: a piece of vivid fiction meant to give the Five Rites an air of Oriental romance in order to encourage potential students to take them seriously.

The value of the Five Rites, however, does not depend on the accuracy of the origin story in Peter Kelder's booklet. Over the eight decades since that book was published, the Rites have proven their worth as a source of health and vitality for people of all ages. What lies behind the facade of Asian wisdom, furthermore, is a story at least as fascinating as any yarn the pseudonymous Colonel Bradford could tell—a story of secret traditions and forgotten lore from many sources that flowed together in late nineteenth and early twentieth century Europe and America, and gave rise to a system of inner transformation in which the Five Rites were central.

In the chapters to come, my first task will be to untangle the various threads that were spun together to create the Five Rites as they appear in Kelder's booklet. My second task will be to follow each of those threads back as far as possible, to reveal something of the landscape of ideas and practices that gave rise to these remarkable exercises. Once those tasks are complete, the final stage of my exploration will be to spin the threads back together, putting the Five Rites in as much of their original context as I can, and describing in detail the practice of the broader system in which the Rites have their place—a system of inner alchemy meant to awaken certain subtle powers of the human body and mind.

The process of tracing a lost occult tradition requires many of the same mental skills that private investigators and police detectives use in their work. The tradition, like the identity or whereabouts of the perpetrator of a crime, is deliberately hidden and has to be reconstructed from whatever fragmentary clues come to hand. A fingerprint here, a scuff mark there, a bit of carpet fiber adhering to the grip of a revolver or the clothing on a corpse: these are the scraps of evidence that allow a detective to focus in on a single suspect. In the same way, a distinctive phrase here, a curious detail of teaching there, a connection between two teachers or schools, can allow the investigator of occult traditions to get past the barriers of secrecy and recover a system of theory and practice that has been lost for decades or centuries.

One of the most important clues in the present case is also one of the most obvious. Kelder titled his work *The Eye of Revelation* and ended his text with a vivid sentence: "Truly, I thought to myself, The Eye of Revelation is upon the world." Nowhere in his booklet does he explain what that Eye is or how it relates to the Five Rites. The Eye of Revelation, as I will show, is a specific anatomical structure in the human brain, and its stimulation through the Rites and certain other practices detailed in the following chapters has potent psychophysical effects on human consciousness and health. The awakening of that Eye was the central secret taught by a number of esoteric societies in late nineteenth and early twentieth century America and Europe. The Five Rites, while they are valid on their own as an exercise system for health, vitality, and longevity, take on a further importance as keys to that awakening. Full instructions for the process are given in this book.

A few words of thanks are in order before we proceed. I am indebted to James Borges, director of the Borderland Sciences Research Association, for access to several important source documents, notably Emile Raux's *Hindu Secrets of Virility and Rejuvenation*, which filled in several crucial details in the history of the Five Rites. I also owe a great deal to two online archives, www.archive.org and www.iapsop.org, which have made an astonishing wealth of classic out-of-copyright occult texts available in PDF formats for free download; without the labor of the individuals who have contributed time and money to both these resources, this book would never have been possible.

The Eye of Revelation began with a narrative, and this book will do the same. We will start searching for the secret of the Five Rites in a setting at least as exotic as any Himalayan lamasery: the Los Angeles occult scene between the two world wars.

CHAPTER 1

The Teacher

Some cities, in some periods of history, are poised more than others on the breaking wave of the future. In 1939, the greater Los Angeles area was one of those places. Hollywood was hitting its stride as the manufacturer and magnet of America's dreams. Cutting-edge industries such as aviation and electronics thrived in the city and the towns around it, drawn by business-friendly policies and a state university system that turned out engineers and researchers at a record pace. Between Tinseltown and technology, extraordinary amounts of money sloshed through the greater LA economy, and the resulting boom made the region a land of opportunity that drew newcomers from far and wide. Among the economic sectors that ended up making its mark on the Los Angeles area was occultism.

The occult traditions of the Western world have a long history. Centuries before the birth of Christ, Greek thinkers such as Pythagoras and Empedocles gathered up the spiritual heritage of ancient Egypt and combined it with the traditional lore of their own culture to create a spirituality that put personal experience of inner realities ahead of formal practices or blind belief in doctrines. Systematized in the heyday of the Roman Empire by the philosophers Iamblichus and Proclus, and also by the mystics and theologians of the Gnostic movement, these teachings were driven underground with the rise of dogmatic Christianity and maintained a hole-and-corner existence all through the Dark Ages that followed.

When the Renaissance weakened the grip of dogma on the European mind, the descendants of those same teachings came boiling up out of hiding. The long years of secrecy had left their mark, not least in the name these teachings went by. Writers in the Renaissance called the teachings "occult philosophy," from the Latin word *occultus*, "hidden." Later on, in the nineteenth century, that phrase was rounded off to "occultism."

Occultism arrived in America in colonial times and had already set down deep roots on American soil long before the Declaration of Independence was signed. During most eras of America's later history, one of the nation's great cities became the most important center of occult teaching and publishing, the place where the most influential occultists gathered and where new understandings of the old secret wisdom blossomed. In colonial times, Philadelphia was the most important occult center in North America; in the first half of the nineteenth century, Boston took on that role; in the latter part of the nineteenth century and the first years of the twentieth, it was Chicago. Through most of the twentieth century, in exactly the same way, Los Angeles was the throbbing heart of American occultism, the place where ancient teachings and new visions collided to shape and reshape the collective imagination of an era.

The first great beachhead of occultism in California was further down the coast at Point Loma near San Diego, where a group of mystics connected to the Theosophical Society founded a commune in 1900. Nine years later Oceanside, also located in the greater San Diego area, became the headquarters of the Rosicrucian Fellowship, a worldwide association of Christian mystics who believe in reincarnation and practice astrology, which will play a significant role in our story as it unfolds. By the time of the First World War, however, Los Angeles had long outstripped its southern rival as an occult hub, and by 1939, San Diego was an occult backwater compared to the thriving esoteric scene further north.

The Theosophical Society, though it had gone through many ups and downs since its founding in 1875, was still the world's most influential occult organization in 1939. It had a big presence in the

Los Angeles area, centered at the Krotona Institute in Beachwood Canyon, just uphill from Hollywood. On Los Feliz Boulevard, the headquarters of the Philosophical Research Society—headed by Manly P. Hall, who would become the grand old man of American occultism in later decades—was under construction during that year. While the bulldozers and backhoes labored, Hall gave his weekly lectures to ample crowds in rented spaces closer in to downtown or went on tour to dazzle audiences in other cities. Two other influential organizations, Guy and Edna Ballard's I Am Activity and Elbert Benjamine's Brotherhood of Light, were both headquartered in Los Angeles at that time, and the city also boasted one of the few American branches of the Hermetic Order of the Golden Dawn, the most prestigious occult secret society in the English-speaking world.

These were the big names. There were hundreds of lesser figures, small fry in the surging ocean of Los Angeles occultism. One of them was Harry J. Gardener, whose Mid-Day Press published the first and second editions of *The Eye of Revelation*.

ೞ

His real name was Henry Lawrence Juhnke, and he was born in the little town of Gardiner, Oregon in 1890, the son of a logger who had immigrated from Germany and his American-born wife.[1] Sometime between 1900 and 1910, according to census records, the Juhnke family moved to Spokane, Washington, where young Harry worked as a harness maker—this was a viable trade in 1910, when most farm equipment was still pulled by horses. Sometime after that, he married a woman named Leora Miller, but they divorced in Santa Cruz, California, in 1917. When the United States went to war that same year, Juhnke registered for the draft, though he apparently was never inducted, and the 1920 census found him back in Santa Cruz, working as a clerk at the local Woolworth's department store.

These faint traces of an ordinary American life give little indication of the deeper aspects of Juhnke's life. According to his autobiographical essay *Money, Magic, and Mystery In My Life*, he had several encounters with strange phenomena in childhood, and his occult training began in his teen years. His mother, a devout Methodist, died when he was fourteen, and his father became a Spiritualist during her final illness

---

[1] I am indebted to research conducted by Marc Demarest and Jerry Watt for the facts of Juhnke's life. See Demarest 2016 and Watt 2022.

and allowed his son to study along with him. Later Juhnke had other uncanny experiences, including prophetic dreams, and grew more and more interested in the occult side of existence.

Occult training was easy to come by in his time, for a remarkably simple reason. Around 1900, the ready availability of cheap duplicating technologies and changes in the postal code kick-started the golden age of American correspondence courses. The back pages of every magazine in America's busy newsstands bristled with ads for study-by-mail courses on every subject imaginable. Occult teachers were quick to recognize the possibilities of the new medium, and by the time Harry Juhnke came of age, plenty of occult schools passed on the wisdom of the ages via weekly or monthly lessons for modest fees.

Whether Juhnke studied one or more of these courses will probably never be known, though it seems likely. What we do know is that in 1924 he began to teach his own course by mail. That was when his first advertisements appear, in the classifieds column of *Popular Science* magazine. He was living in Sacramento at that time, but by 1930, he had relocated to Los Angeles, where he spent the rest of his life, and was using the name Harry J. Gardener. Why he changed his name is uncertain, though the slang term "junkie" had entered common American usage by then and he may have gotten tired of having his name confused with that label.

In that year, according to census records, he lived in the men's dormitory at the Bible Institute of Los Angeles at the corner of 6th and Hope in downtown Los Angeles. The Bible Institute was a huge building thirteen stories tall that took up most of a city block. Its twin neon signs, reading JESUS SAVES, were familiar landmarks to Los Angeles residents from the time of the First World War until the building was demolished in 1988. Founded and funded by Lyman Stewart, longtime president of Union Oil Company of California, it offered free training for Protestant missionaries and ministers. The dormitories were exclusively for students, so Gardener (as we may as well call him from this point on) must have enrolled in the Bible Institute and studied there.

Within a few years of his relocation to Los Angeles, however, he began publishing his own spiritual teachings in booklet form, and these had very little in common with ordinary Protestant Christianity. The first of what would become his core series of lessons, *Outwitting Tomorrow*, appeared in 1934. He called his lessons monographs, which may point to one of the inspirations of his teachings—the Ancient Mystical Order Rosae Crucis (AMORC), an influential Rosicrucian order which has its American headquarters further up the California coast in San Jose, uses the same term for its correspondence lessons. *Outwitting Tomorrow* became the introduction to his system and was followed by more than sixty monographs as well as a booklet of predictions titled *What's Next?* issued annually from 1938 until 1967.

Gardener's spiritual teachings are classic twentieth century American popular occultism, focusing on what he called the Five-Fold Life—the attainment of spiritual, mental, social, physical, and financial success. He believed that the world would enter the Age of Aquarius in the year 2000, ushering in an age of peace and plenty, but that most of humanity would perish in a cascade of disasters before then, leaving only the elect to enter into the Seventh Millennium. (It needs to be said that most of his predictions were just as inaccurate as this one; prophecy was not Gardener's strong suit.) Most people, he taught, were mass-minded, with their twelve mental activities frozen in negative states. Those who began to shake themselves free of mass-mindedness and make some of their mental activities positive became "budding individuals," and if they persevered, they would become Individuals and then Masters.

Since the Age of Aquarius was an age of youth, Gardener considered "youthening" practices to be important parts of the work of becoming a budding individual and devoted several of his own books to explaining how to overcome the aging process and become young and fit again at any age. His instructions for doing this, and more generally for making the twelve mental activities positive and attuning to the rising currents of the Aquarian age, are refreshingly straightforward and practical when compared to some of the other occult teachings of the time, and he included a great many exercises and practices in his writings—something many other occult teachers of the time never got around to doing. His monographs therefore found plenty of readers.

The monographs and his many other publications, amounting to some 140 titles in all, were published by Gardener's own press, which was located for many years at 1044 South Olive Street in Los Angeles. Under various names—the Mid-Day Press, the New Era Press, the Golden Dawn Press, and others—his firm mostly issued Gardener's own books and pamphlets, but Gardener also published books under other bylines: Elizabeth McElroy Binder, James C. Hollenbeck, F. M. J. Smythe, and, of course, Peter Kelder. His publications also included titles under the pseudonyms Frater VIII°, Frater IX°, Frater XII°, and The Magus.[2] Frater VIII° was Gardener himself (several of his books appear in some editions under this name); the identities of the others remain unknown for the time being.

Some people spend their lives seeking a successful niche. Others achieve one and settle comfortably into it for the rest of their time on the planet. Harry J. Gardener belonged to the second category. He spent the rest of a tolerably long life in Los Angeles, publishing and selling his monographs and his annual volumes of prophecy. What else he might have done awaits the attention of researchers willing to chase down clues in Los Angeles-area records. He died in 1969 and is buried at Forest Lawn Park in Hollywood. His teachings still have an active following today, though they have not achieved the worldwide attention of the Five Rites.

CB

Read *The Eye of Revelation* alongside the writings of Harry J. Gardener and it's impossible to avoid noticing that quite a bit of the text must have been written by Gardener himself. This is not simply a matter of prose style, though *The Eye of Revelation* does read like one of Gardener's monographs. The narrative of *The Eye of Revelation*—the dialog between the author and the knowledgeable Colonel Bradford—uses one of Gardener's classic frames for communicating his teachings.

In *Outwitting Tomorrow*, for example, the frame narrative for the book is a series of conversations between an ordinary middle-aged man, John Workman, and the mysterious Mr. Grayson, who instructs Workman in a set of secret teachings that free him from the burdens of age and show him how to face life with new enthusiasm. Replace Workman with Peter Kelder and Mr. Grayson with Colonel Bradford and you have essentially the same story. Fictional accounts of monasteries in which very old monks have strength and vitality that puts younger men to shame also feature in several of Gardener's books, including *The Secret Science of Life*, published in 1942. The narrative

---

[2] Gardener's publications often include sections under the bylines of other Fraters; for example, *Outwitting Tomorrow* has sections credited to Frater IX° and Frater XII°, and The Golden Gate to the Garden of Allah has a section by Frater III°.

that introduces the teachings in *The Eye of Revelation* is very clearly cut from the same cloth.

There is also a significant amount of shared content uniting *The Eye of Revelation* with Harry Gardener's other publications. One of the health rules included in the book—the practice of drinking raw egg yolks—appears in Gardener's *Outwitting Tomorrow*, published five years before the first edition of *The Eye of Revelation*. Another teaching in the book, the practice of rubbing butter into the scalp to reverse hair loss, is set out in much more detail in a book Gardener published in 1944, *Fire, Air, Water, and Earth* by F.M.J. Smythe. Still another, the injunction to avoid speaking in a high-pitched "old man's voice," is found in Gardener's 1942 volume *Turn Back The Years*.

The dietary rules set out in *The Eye of Revelation* also come from a non-Tibetan source, though it's not a source with any unique connection to Harry J. Gardener. Part Three of Kelder's book is a brief summary of the Hay diet, the most popular alternative dietary theory in early twentieth century America. Created by William Howard Hay, M.D. on the basis of what was then state-of-the-art research on digestion, the Hay diet—also known as "food combining"—set out three categories of foods: protein foods, starch foods, and neutral foods. Protein foods and starch foods, according to the Hay diet, should never be eaten at the same time, though either one can be eaten with neutral foods.[3]

This is the same system *The Eye of Revelation* presents. Hay's own books add a great many complexities to the system, but in occult schools and correspondence courses of the time, these were usually left out, leaving a simplified version like the one found in Kelder's book. It's unlikely, to use no stronger term, that lamas in a distant monastery in the Himalayas were up to date on the latest popular health fads in the United States, much less the modifications of those fads common in American occult circles in 1939. This is another piece of evidence that the story of Colonel Bradford and the lamas was a work of fiction, like Gardener's story of John Workman and Mr. Grayson, rather than an actual account of the origins of the Rites.

Yet the presence of the Hay diet in *The Eye of Revelation* has another clue to offer. While I have not been able to locate and read copies of all Harry Gardener's books and pamphlets on life extension and

---

[3] See, for example, Hay 1929.

"youthening," none of those I have studied refers to the Hay diet or anything like it. The focus of Gardener's teachings was always on the mind. He recommended adding raw egg yolks, fresh fruit, buttermilk and a mixture of honey and fresh butter to the diet, and avoiding alcohol, sugar, white bread, and white potatoes, but changes in attitude and instructions on how to think positively rather than negatively form the core of Gardener's teachings.

A good example is his *Five Fold Life Extension Course*, an 18-lesson course from 1957 that summarizes his system. It includes not a single exercise or dietary rule. Its only physical practice is a method of relaxation, and its teachings focus on cultivating positive emotions and developing the mind's capacities to release tension and concentrate its energies. Elsewhere in his writings, he includes a certain number of breathing exercises and one exercise that combine breathing and movement, but these play secondary roles in his system, and they are very easy compared to the body-core workout of the Five Rites.

Gardener may well have written or co-written *The Eye of Revelation*, in other words, but there is no evidence that he was responsible for the Five Rites or the rest of the pamphlet's unique content. He never advertised *The Eye of Revelation* along with his other books, nor did he copyright it in his own name or in that of one of his presses, as he usually did. It's thus far more likely than not that Peter Kelder (or whoever wrote under that pseudonym) and Harry J. Gardener were two different people, though Gardener wrote a great deal of the text in Kelder's book. This sort of arrangement was tolerably common in the 1930s. Iconic weird-fantasy writer H.P. Lovecraft, to cite only one famous name, made much of his living in that decade by revising and rewriting stories for paying clients, who then published the stories under their own names.

One possibility well worth investigating, given the general character of the Los Angeles occult scene at the time *The Eye of Revelation* first saw print, is that Gardener and Kelder belonged to the same occult society. Gardener's pen name Frater VIII° strongly suggests this, since "Frater" (Latin for "brother") was a common term for members of such a society, especially one connected to the Rosicrucian movement.

Some connection between Gardener's work and the Rosicrucian tradition clearly existed: Gardener's monograph #26, "The Rose-Cross Clan," focuses on Rosicrucian symbolism and identifies the material he teaches with the Rosicrucian current. (We will be discussing the Rosicrucians and their complex heritage later on, in Chapter Five.) Since some of Gardener's books were published under the label of The Golden Dawn Press, it is just possible that this society had some connection to the Hermetic Order of the Golden Dawn, the prestigious occult society mentioned earlier, which also had Rosicrucian connections; it has to be admitted, however, that none of the material in Gardener's writings has any obvious connection to the recorded teachings of the Golden Dawn.

If an occult society lies behind the hints dropped by Gardener, Frater III°, Frater IX°, and Frater XII° would likely have been other members of the society, and The Magus may have been its head—the title Magus (Latin for "magician") was one of the standard terms for the presiding officer of a Rosicrucian society. It is quite possible that these pseudonyms concealed some of the other writers known to have published books with Gardener, though further research will be needed to sort this out. One clue worth following up is the seal of the organization, which appears in many of Gardener's publications in the 1940s and 1950s: a pentagram representing the Five-Fold Life intertwined with a circle symbolizing silence, and inside both a triangle standing for the three principles of Zeal, Fervor, and Enthusiasm.

Though it seems very likely that Gardener and Kelder belonged to the same small occult society, one of dozens in 1930s Los Angeles, conclusive evidence one way or another has not yet surfaced. It can be demonstrated beyond question, however, that one or both of them had connections in the wider world of American occultism and drew on those connections in the process of writing *The Eye of Revelation*.

The evidence here is quite straightforward. Kelder's book was not the first appearance in print of the Five Rites and the distinctive system of seven vortices that the Rites are meant to awaken. It is, however, the first place where all five of the Rites and the system of vortices appear together. The First Rite, the remaining four Rites, and the vortices saw print in three different volumes before the first edition of *The Eye of Revelation* was published. Each of these sources has a complex story behind it. Taken together, they reveal a broader landscape of mind-body practices that gave rise to the Five Rites, but they also point to a tradition that goes far beyond the material in Kelder's booklet—a tradition this book will attempt to reveal.

CHAPTER 2

The Exercises

The quest for the sources of Kelder's work takes us first to another nearly forgotten booklet published in 1939, the same year as the first edition of *The Eye of Revelation*. Its title is *Hindu Secrets of Vitality and Rejuvenation*, and it was issued by the Basic Science Fellowship, another small publisher based in Denver, Colorado. What makes it relevant to our theme is that it teaches a set of four exercises that are nearly identical with the last four of the Five Rites.

The byline on the cover of the booklet is Emile Raux, but once again we are dealing with a pseudonym. The figure behind "Emile Raux" was Charles B. Roth, who was in the same business as Harry J. Gardener—that is, he was a prolific author of self-published books and pamphlets, sold mostly by mail. Roth's specific focus was a little different from Gardener's. He wrote books on salesmanship, some of which are still in print today, and also a series of booklets on health-related topics, including the one we are discussing.

Hindu Secrets, as we will call Roth's booklet for convenience, is by no means identical to *The Eye of Revelation*. Its focus is on male sexual virility, not on health or rejuvenation in any more general sense. Postal regulations in 1939 made it impossible for Roth to use the words "penis" or "erection" in his pamphlet, but he gave the English language a good workout in order to talk about the subject of male potency in every way he legally could. That, in turn, is the be-all and end-all of the four exercises Roth teaches; spirituality has no place in the text, nor do any of the rejuvenating habits Peter Kelder and Harry Gardener put in their booklet, with one curious exception: the habit of washing in cool but not cold water after practicing the exercises is in Roth's text as well.

Copyright data offers a useful clue to the relation between Roth's booklet and Gardener's. *Hindu Secrets* was copyrighted on February 23, 1939. *The Eye of Revelation* was copyrighted on December 1 of the same year. Gardener's booklet is listed in the copyright records as "copyrighted following publication," so it could have been published at any point during 1939. Most likely, however, given the copyright date on Roth's work, Gardener's was published some time afterward, and some researchers—including the editor of a recent reprint of *Hindu Secrets*—have assumed on this basis that Gardener simply plagiarized Roth's book.

The situation is hardly as simple as that, however. Roth's exercises are not quite identical to Kelder's; the differences are modest but significant. Roth gives only four of the Rites, and he gives them in a different order. His first movement is the Fifth Rite of Kelder's book, his second is the Fourth Rite, his third is the Second Rite, and his fourth is the Third Rite.

Furthermore, Roth apparently knows nothing of the seven vortices central to the Five Rites of *The Eye of Revelation*. His exercises are meant to stimulate the endocrine glands into activity, rather than to awaken vortices into new life. Since the purpose of Roth's exercises is masculine virility, he focuses attention on the glands central to male sexual performance—the testes, the prostate, and the tiny Cowper's glands—though he also mentions the adrenal, thyroid, thymus, and pituitary glands.

In addition, Roth refers to the exercises not as Rites but as *dands*. This is a Hindi word, the proper name of an exercise similar to the Fifth Rite, which has been practiced by Indian wrestlers since ancient times. (Many physical fitness buffs in the Western world nowadays know *dands* as "Indian pushups.") This is part of a frame that assigns Roth's system to a Hindu origin, rather than tracing it to lamas and thus to Himalayan Buddhist sources. It is worth noting that Roth didn't offer any explanation of the way he came into possession of a secret exercise system otherwise reserved for Hindus of the higher castes; there is no equivalent of the Colonel Bradford story in *Hindu Secrets*. There is simply a flat assertion that the exercises Roth taught had this origin.

The difference between the two origin stories makes more of a difference than many Western people realize. Hinduism and Buddhism are related in much the same way as Judaism and Christianity. Hinduism is by far the older of the two, and Buddhism shares some of its basic ideas, but rejected other core Hindu concepts in the process of breaking away and establishing itself as an independent faith. The richly developed yoga traditions of Hinduism have equivalents in Buddhism, but Hindu and Buddhist yogas are by and large far from identical. The one thing they have in common, of course, is that in America in 1939, both Hinduism and Buddhism were pleasantly exotic and were put to work by American spiritual teachers in their advertising.

An equivalent project well worth keeping in mind as we proceed was the 1905 book *Hatha Yoga, or the Yogi Philosophy of Physical Well-Being*. The byline on the title page was Yogi Ramacharaka, but we are once again in pseudonym territory: the author's real name was William Walker Atkinson, one of the most prolific and successful figures in the alternative spirituality movement of the time, and an even more enthusiastic fan of pen names than the writers we've already discussed. (He was also Theron Q. Dumont and all three of the Three Initiates who are credited with writing *The Kybalion*, one of the enduring classics of American occultism.)

In *Hatha Yoga*, Atkinson taught a set of movement exercises that he claimed came straight out of Hindu yoga. What makes this fascinating in the context of our exploration is that with one exception, which will be discussed shortly, the exercises that Atkinson taught had nothing in common with yoga, or for that matter any other form of Asian exercises. They were Western calisthenics pure and simple, of the sort that could be found in plenty of less colorfully titled books on exercise published in America at the same time. Trace their lineage back further and it leads not to India but to Germany.

cs

Physical exercise is doubtless as old as the first cities. People in rural settings, whether they make their livings as hunter-gatherers, herders, or farmers, get plenty of physical exercise in the course of their daily activities. Once the first urban centers rose and made sedentary lifestyles possible, however, physical weakness and illness caused by inadequate muscular effort must have followed within a generation or so. Some bright soul in a forgotten mud-brick town thousands of years ago met the resulting need by coming up with the first exercise routine.

For complex reasons rooted in religious attitudes toward the human body, however, Europe entered the modern era without its own traditions of exercise. Europeans who wanted vigorous movement could play sports, take up martial arts such as boxing and fencing, or engage in other vigorous activities, but the idea of exercise for its own sake had gotten lost somewhere in the Dark Ages and had to be reintroduced from abroad.

This was accomplished by a French Jesuit missionary, Joseph-Marie Amiot, with his essay *Notice du Cong-Fou des Bonzes Tao-sée* (*Notes on the Kung-fu of the Taoist Monks*), published in Paris in 1779. The postures and movements that Père Amiot described, and illustrated with quaint copperplate engravings, came from qigong, the traditional Chinese system of health exercises. They sparked a great deal of interest in exercise among physicians and the general public over the decades that followed.

That interest had its greatest impact further east, in Germany and Scandinavia. In 1793, German educator J.C.F. GutsMuths published the first modern book on gymnastics, *Gymnastik für die Jugend* (*Gymnastics for Youth*), and kick-started a continent-wide fad for gymnastic exercise. In 1810, Friedrich Jahn, another German educator, began teaching gymnastics to his pupils and soon found himself with a mass movement on his hands. Germany in those days was still a chaos of little countries at the mercy of their more powerful neighbors. In 1810, that meant above all France's Emperor Napoleon I, whose armies had by then been marching back and forth across the German landscape for most of a decade.

Jahn saw gymnastic exercise as a way to inspire Germany's youth with courage and patriotic fervor. Plenty of German youths were more than willing to listen. When the German kingdoms rose in revolt against Napoleon in 1813, Jahn raised a volunteer force from among his gymnastic students, and he and they served with distinction in the war that followed. From that point on, Jahn—"Father Jahn" to generations of German athletes thereafter—became the iconic head of the *Turnverein* or Gymnastics League and helped spark a gymnastics craze that spread across Europe and also inspired young athletes in the United States.

Jahn's movement was not without competition. In 1814, Swedish writer Per Henrik Ling founded a school of exercise in Stockholm and created modern calisthenics. Where Jahn's gymnastics relied on exercise apparatus—vaulting horses, balance beams, rings suspended from ropes, and the like—Ling's exercises were performed without equipment, using vigorous movements and body weight. His system also found plenty of enthusiastic practitioners, and for some decades proponents of gymnastics and calisthenics sniped at one another in the letters columns of newspapers and magazines, the nineteenth century equivalent of internet forums.

Read books on the two systems, or watch videos of old-fashioned gymnastics and calisthenics in action, and one curious common factor is hard to miss. Practitioners of both systems were taught to exercise their arms and legs while holding their bodies stiff. To a modern eye, there is something very strange about the illustrations from nineteenth century exercise books, which show young men working out while their bodies from shoulders to hips remain as rigid as bricks. Weird as it seems now, that was how Europeans held their bodies for many centuries. From the stiff doublets of the Renaissance to the stiff waistcoats of the Victorians, and of course the even stiffer corsets worn by women all through the same period, holding the torso absolutely rigid was standard for any respectable person. It's no wonder that constipation was a serious public health problem all through that period—people routinely died of it—and equally unsurprising that so many Europeans at that time found the free bodily movement of people from other cultures at once so shocking and so tempting.

Most of the "hatha yoga" exercises included in the book by William Walker Atkinson mentioned above come straight out of Ling's tradition of calisthenics. The practitioner moves arms and legs or at most tilts the stiff torso forward, backward, or to the sides, using the hips as the fulcrum. The one exception—and it is at the end of Atkinson's list, as though tacked on at the last minute—is a set of movements with a fascinating and revealing similarity to the last four of the Five Rites. Here is Atkinson's description:

Exercise XI

(1) Lie upon your stomach, extending your arms above your head and then bowed upward, and your legs stretched out full length and raised backward and upward. The correct position may be carried in

the mind by imagining a watch-crystal or a saucer resting on the table on its middle, with both ends turning upward. (2) Lower and raise the arms and legs, several times. (3) Then, turn over on your back, and lie extended at full length, with arms extended straight out, upward over the head, with back of fingers touching the ground. (4) Then raise up both legs from the waist until they stand straight up in the air, like the mast of a ship, your upper body and arms remaining in the last position named. Lower the legs and raise them several times. (5) Resume position 3, lying flat upon the back at full length with arms extended straight out upward, over the head, with backs of fingers touching the ground; (6) Then gradually raise body to sitting position, with arms projecting straight out in front of the shoulders. Then go back gradually to the lying-down position, and repeat the rising and lowering several times. (7) Then turn over on the face and stomach again, and assume the following position: Keeping the body rigid from head to foot, raise your body until its weight rests upon your palms (the arms being stretched out straight in front of you) at one end, and upon your toes at the other end. Then gradually bend arms at the elbow, allowing your chest to sink to the floor; then raise up your chest and upper body by straightening out your arms, the entire weight falling upon the arms, with the toes as a pivot—this last is a difficult motion and should not be overdone at first.

The rigid torso of the European tradition has begun to break down. Atkinson's exercise works the spine forward and backward, arching the back in the first two steps, and then exercising the abdominal and hip muscles in the next four. He finishes up with a stiff-bodied pushup, as though to atone for the flexibility of the earlier movements. Practice the movements of Exercise XI a few times and compare them to the Five Rites, and it may occur to you that the final movement can be transformed quite readily into the Fifth Rite, and the remaining movements look like rough drafts of the Second and Fourth Rites.

It is by no means impossible that this is exactly what they are. Atkinson was among the most successful and widely read writers in the American occult scene at the dawn of the twentieth century. His teachings were picked up and reworked in various directions by a great many occultists in North America and elsewhere over the decades that followed. This is standard practice in the occult community. The claims made by some occult groups about ancient secrets passed down unchanged since the beginning of time are pure window dressing. In reality, most occultists are inveterate tinkerers, trying endless variations on their rituals and practices to see if they can get better results with this or that change. Thus it's plausible that Exercise XI might have been taken up by occultists and reworked in various ways, with the closely related exercises published by Roth and Kelder among the results.

A further line of evidence supports this suggestion. The occult community, after all, is far from the only American subculture that likes to tinker with practices. The physical fitness scene is just as enthusiastic in this regard. Thus it may be relevant that the first ten exercises of Atkinson's supposed "hatha yoga," the movements that follow Ling's stiff-body pattern, were taken up by American football star and exercise maven Walter Camp. Reworked by him, they were publicized heavily in 1918 as "the Daily Dozen," a set of calisthenics that became hugely popular across America between the two world wars. Camp was careful not to mention his source—then as now, occultism has a whiff of scandal about it—but a comparison of Atkinson's exercises with Camp's Daily Dozen shows the line of descent clearly enough.

One additional exercise connected with our inquiry is worth mentioning here. This is the Rising Call, which appears at several points in the writings of Harry J. Gardener. The version I give here is from his 1936 manual of practice *Streamline Minds*:

> The exercise is as follows: Standing erect, place the right thumb against the right nostril, allowing the fingers of the hand to extend upward in-line with the forehead. Now through the left nostril completely fill the lungs with air. Then with the index finger of the same hand close the left nostril also.
>
> With the lungs filled and the lips partly open so that there will be no pressure in the mouth, bend over from the waist, getting the head lowered as far as is conveniently possible. Then allow a portion of the air in the lungs to gently come back into the nose so as to create just a very slight pressure there. This position allows the blood to flow into every part of the brain which, along with the air in the lungs, has a very energizing effect upon the entire system and especially upon the sensitive nerve centers of the brain.
>
> When the desire to resume breathing is quite strong, rise to the erect position, then close the left nostril and allow the breath to escape through the right nostril by removing thumb. Do not force it out with great speed; nor should you retard it to any great extent. Just let it flow out freely and naturally until the lungs are emptied without forcing out the last particle of air through sheer force.

Now, with positively no intervening breaths—in other words, with the very next inhalation of air—repeat the process. Close the right nostril with the right thumb; inhale through the left nostril; close both nostrils; bend over until ready to exhale; then stand erect; remove the thumb from the right nostril and exhale. Do this three times. That is, you fill the lungs three times, you hold the breath and bend over three times, and you exhale three times.[1]

Once again, the body is being flexed, in the same way that several of the Five Rites flex it—though in a much less strenuous manner. It took time, and probably a great deal of experimentation, for first explorations such as the Rising Call and Atkinson's Exercise XI to give rise to the robust flexing of the Five Rites.

ભ

It's worth taking a moment at this point to go into more detail about the relationship between the exercises we have been discussing and the traditions of yoga. Peter Kelder and Charles B. Roth both traced their respective exercises back to the Indian subcontinent, though as already noted they disagreed on the details, and most research into the Five Rites since their time has focused on finding some Indian or Tibetan source for the exercises. That was a direction worth exploring, and it turned up some fascinating if equivocal findings.

There is one exercise in the tradition we are considering that definitely comes from an Indian source. This is the Sixth Rite in Kelder's book. In yoga practice, it is called *uddiyana bandha*, and it is done precisely the way Kelder describes. Not only that, it has the effect Kelder assigns to it—Swami Sivananda's classic manual *Kundalini Yoga* notes that "[t]his exercise helps a lot in keeping up Brahmacharya (i.e., celibacy)."[2] *Uddiyana bandha*, however, was one of the earliest yoga exercises transmitted to the West, partly because it is quite easy to perform even by Westerners with inflexible bodies, and partly because sexual purity was so heavily valued in late nineteenth- and early twentieth century Western societies. By the time *The Eye of Revelation* saw print, the technique of *uddiyana bandha* and its connection to celibacy were both well known in Western occult circles.

---

[1] Gardener 1936, p. 4.
[2] Sivananda 1980, p. 136.

The other exercises are much less easy to trace to Asian originals. Kelder's Fifth Rite and Roth's first *dand*, as already noted, have a close equivalent in the classic Indian *dand*, one of the traditional exercises practiced relentlessly by Indian wrestlers since time out of mind. In India, however, the *dand* is invariably paired with the *bethak*, a deep squat performed with feet placed well apart, combined with a swinging movement of the arms; there is of course no equivalent of the *bethak* in either of the two booklets we are discussing. In Indian practice, furthermore, the *dand* has a range of subtle details that do not appear in either booklet's version. Kelder's and Roth's exercises, to be frank, look like instructions for performing a classic *dand* written by someone who had never witnessed one but had simply read a description in a book or magazine and tried to imitate it.

The same point could be made just as accurately of the Third Rite of Kelder's booklet and the fourth *dand* of Roth's. This is similar to one of the classic *asanas* of Indian hatha yoga, *Ustrasana* or camel pose. Once again, however, the exercises from the booklets resemble nothing so much as a camel pose done by someone who had read about it in a book.

It is quite possible, again, that this is exactly what happened. Yoga schools are so ubiquitous in the Western world these days that it can be hard to remember just how difficult it was for people in Western countries, not much more than half a century ago, to get any sort of accurate instruction in hatha yoga. While there were several previous attempts to bring yoga to the West, the first successful hatha yoga school in North America was founded by Indra Devi (another pseudonym— her real name was Eugenie Peterson) in Hollywood in 1947.

It was only after then that hatha yoga began to transform itself from an exotic teaching from the far side of the world to a normal part of life for tens of millions of people in most Western countries. Before then, people in the West who were interested in hatha yoga either had to travel to India to study it or made do with books and magazine articles of extremely mixed quality, illustrated with photos or line drawings of equally varied accuracy.

Certain elements of yoga practice, to be sure, found their way into the West very early on. The Theosophist William Quan Judge published a workable English translation of the *Yoga Sutras* of Patanjali in 1889, and Aleister Crowley's *Eight Lectures on Yoga*—largely based on Patanjali's work, though it gave instructions for a set of asanas Crowley seems to have made up out of whole cloth—first saw print in 1939. As the popularity of Atkinson's mistitled book *Hatha Yoga* demonstrates, however, the reading public in the early twentieth century knew next to nothing about the physical dimension of hatha yoga. That made it easy for Roth to assign his version of the exercises to a Hindu source, and for Kelder to make use of Americans' even more complete ignorance of Tibetan practices to assign his version of the exercises to a collection of otherwise untraceable Himalayan lamas.

One of the first significant breakthroughs in the transmission of Indian exercises in the West, however, came in 1936. In that year Bhavanarao Pant Pratinidhi, the Rajah of Aundh, came to England to promote a traditional Indian exercise he had practiced for many years, the *Surya Namaskar* or Sun Salutation.[3] These days *Surya Namaskar* is very often taught as part of hatha yoga, but at that time it was considered wholly separate—it did not find its way into the standard hatha yoga curriculum until the 1950s, when yoga teacher Swami Sivananda played a central role in popularizing it in Britain and the English-speaking world generally. Until then, Indian teachers of hatha yoga and *Surya Namaskar* sniped at each other in much the same spirit that partisans of Jahn and Lind had done not so long before.

Bhavanarao wasn't interested in polemic, however. Sixty-seven years old, he was supple and fit, and credited *Surya Namaskar* with that fact; he wanted to share the exercise with as many people as possible, in the West as well as in India. His lectures, and a film he had made showing people doing *Surya Namaskar*, won him an interview with English journalist Louise Morgan and a series of instructional articles in the *News Chronicle*, one of the popular newspapers of the day. An instructional book on *Surya Namaskar* issued by a British mass market publisher, *The Ten-Point Way to Health*, followed in 1938, written by Bhavanarao with Morgan's help, and it remained in print for more than three decades thereafter.

This detail of the history of yoga may have more relevance to the emergence of the Five Rites than it might seem at first glance. To begin with, *Surya Namaskar* contains the distinctive postures of the Fifth Rite, and in the form taught in *The Ten-Point Way to Health*, the details of those movements have more in common with those of the Fifth Rite

---

[3] See Goldberg 2016, pp. 180–335, for the history of the transmission of *Surya Namaskar* to the West.

than the classic Indian *dand* does. *Surya Namaskar* is also a sequence of movements, as the Five Rites are, rather than a set of static poses like those of hatha yoga. Perhaps more important is the way that *The Ten-Point Way to Health* reframed *Surya Namaskar* as a health and longevity exercise.

As Elliott Goldberg points out in his history *The Path of Modern Yoga*, neither hatha yoga nor *Surya Namaskar* started out with that focus. These exercises were originally used to prepare the body for long sessions of meditation, and it took Indian teachers decades of what could impolitely but accurately be called market research to find out how best to pitch their art to curious but clueless Westerners. Louise Morgan's articles on *Surya Namaskar* played an important role in that process, introducing a yoga-like exercise to a mostly female audience as a way to maintain good health, fitness, and beauty into old age.

That focus on longevity, of course, was also central to Peter Kelder's presentation of the Five Rites in *The Eye of Revelation*. It is at least possible that *The Ten-Point Way to Health* helped inspire Kelder and Roth to write their respective booklets, and just as possible that the book or the earlier newspaper articles gave members of the British and American occult communities some of the ideas that went into the creation of the last four Rites. Under the circumstances, it is unlikely that any conclusive evidence can be found.

One point strongly suggested by the differences between the exercises we have been studying, however, is that they had been in circulation for some time before Kelder and Roth went to work on their booklets. Exercises, especially when they aren't fixed by way of text or images, tend to vary over time as different practitioners adapt them to their own bodies' needs. If Atkinson's Exercise XI had become the starting point for experimentation in the American occult scene as soon as it appeared in 1905, and pictures and descriptions of hatha yoga postures and *Surya Namaskar* in popular media and books helped provide that process with raw material in the years that followed, the closely related but divergent exercises presented by Kelder and Roth would be likely results. Whether that is what happened, certainly, the exercises themselves make sense if understood in those terms.

The differences in intention between Roth's and Kelder's versions of the exercises also make that same point. Both have the goal of restoring vitality and good health to the elderly, but Roth's pamphlet begins and ends there, with a narrow focus on sexual performance. Kelder's pamphlet, by contrast, presents the Five Rites as an exercise system that can be done for health reasons alone but has other dimensions as well. In these two pamphlets, we can catch glimpses of a forgotten subculture at work, taking a set of exercises originally developed for spiritual purposes and making use of them for their health benefits. That same trajectory marks out the history of hatha yoga in the West, so it would be no surprise if the same thing happened with the early forms of the Five Rites.

CHAPTER 3

The Currents

The last four of the Five Rites are thus accounted for, at least to some degree. The First Rite is another matter. It does not appear in Charles B. Roth's booklet, nor can it be traced to the busy pen of William Walker Atkinson or to Western publications about the exercise traditions of the Indian subcontinent. *The Eye of Revelation* compares the First Rite to the turning practice of the Mawlawiyya or Mevlevi Sufis, the so-called whirling dervishes, but the similarity between these practices is more apparent than real: the Mevlevis pivot on the ball of the left foot, using sweeping steps with the right foot to drive the turning motion, and their arms are held in various positions, not straight out as in the First Rite.

As with the rest of the Rites, the First Rite is not Asian in origin. It belongs to a distinct tradition in American occultism and metaphysical thought, one that has left even sparser traces—but the traces can still be followed. Our evidence is yet another forgotten booklet from a small American press.

In 1892, a local publishing house in Minneapolis published a 32-page booklet by the Spiritualist medium Abby A. Judson titled *Development of Mediumship by Terrestrial Magnetism*. Judson, the heretic daughter of a famous Christian missionary, was a professional trance medium and teacher of mediums, moderately well known among Spiritualists in the Midwest. Her booklet taught a method of Spiritualist development that differed sharply from the usual approach. Where other novice Spiritualists simply sat in quiet rooms and with their eyes closed and concentrated on emptying their minds, waiting for the spirits to speak through them, Judson taught her pupils a set of five exercises. They were not the Five Rites and have no resemblance at all to four of the Rites, but they cast a fascinating light back into the origins of the First Rite and forward to one of their lost secrets.

Judson's exercises were intended to work with the animal magnetism that flows through the Earth. She describes them neatly as follows.

1. UNWRAPPING—Face north and then turn clear round and round to the left a few times, eyes open, hands open, palms down, making motions with the arms, as if you were reaching up and out for something and then drawing it toward you. Revolving to the left throws off the currents.
2. RECEIVING THE CURRENTS—On facing the south, stand, heels together, resting on the balls of the feet, eyes closed, head a little bowed, hands stretched to the south, palms down, fingers a little apart. After receiving, shut your hands and turn to the right, to the north.
3. ASKING FOR GOOD INFLUENCES—With eyes open and hands raised, turn round slowly once to the right, feeling and saying the following: "In the name of Infinite Good, in which I live and move and have my being, I beseech all good, pure, true, and loving influences to come to me at this time."
4. WRAPPING UP—Turn clear round and round to the right a few times, eyes open, making exactly the same motions with the arms as in No. 1, the only difference being that you are now turning to the right.
5. LOCKING UP—Pass the positive or warmer hand across the palm of the negative or cooler hand, without touching, two or three times, and then reverse the process.[1]

Her booklet gives a few more details for practitioners. The first, unwrapping movement makes three and a half rotations, beginning

---

[1] Judson 1891, p. 23.

facing north and ending facing south. The fourth, similarly, makes four and a half rotations, again beginning facing north and ending facing south. In the third exercise, the practitioner can invoke positive influences using any wording he or she wishes—Judson's invocation is simply what she herself said while practicing the exercises.

These exercises were not Judson's own invention. According to her writings, she was taught them by her teacher, Dr. H. W. Abbott, another noted Spiritualist of the time. She claims that he got them from a spirit named Osseweago, a king of lost Atlantis who reigned around 14,500 BC. I suspect, for whatever this is worth, that Dr. Abbott was pulling Miss Judson's leg; the name Osseweago sounds rather suspiciously like Oswego, the name of a city in upstate New York, in a region famous for its Spiritualist activities. Oswego is only fifty miles by road from Hydesville, where Spiritualism got its start in 1848, and it was the site of several notable séances and other events in the early history of Spiritualism.

The central reason I doubt Dr. Abbott's seriousness is that the exercise he taught to Judson was framed in the terminology of a tradition rather more recent than ancient Atlantis. The Spiritualist movement in which they both were active drew extensively on the work of Franz Anton Mesmer and his followers, and in particular from a distinctive branch of that tradition that spread from Europe to North America in the middle of the nineteenth century.

cs

These days Mesmer is remembered, if at all, as the inventor of hypnotism. His actual discoveries were considerably more interesting, but they stray into an area of research that has been taboo among scholars and scientists in the mainstream for more than two centuries. Like many other researchers since his time, Mesmer had the great misfortune to notice something that the scientific community in his time and ours insists does not, cannot, and must not exist. That is to say, he discovered the life force.

Nearly every culture around the world and throughout history has had the concept of a life force, an influence or energy that is responsible for the phenomena of biological life, and nearly every human language has a word for that force. It is *prana* in Sanskrit, *qi* in Chinese, *ki* in Japanese, *ruach* in Hebrew, *ruh* in Arabic, *spiritus* in Latin, *ni* in Lakota, *orenda* in Iroquois, and so on through the roster of the world's languages. As far as I know, the only cultures and languages anywhere that lack a common concept and a frequently used word for the life force are those of the modern industrial West.

Two details of history make this lack particularly striking. The first is that European cultures had a word for it until early modern times. The Latin word *spiritus*, the source of the English word "spirit," was the common term for the life force in most of Europe until after the Renaissance. Only with the emergence of modern materialist ideology, with its dogmatic insistence that nothing is real except dead matter, did the concept of the life force drop out of common use, leaving "spirit" and its cognates in other European languages as vague labels for something that isn't matter.

The second detail of history worth noting here is that all through modern times, scholars and scientists in the Western world have kept on rediscovering the life force and giving new names to it. Since the life force has been taboo in scientific circles for more than two hundred years, those scholars and scientists who discover it have invariably been driven out to the fringes, and they and their work make up a substantial chapter in the history of rejected knowledge and alternative research in modern times.[2] That was what happened to Franz Anton Mesmer.

Born in Switzerland in 1734 and educated at a the University of Vienna's prestigious medical school, Mesmer became convinced, as a result of his experiments with patients, that the life force was the missing factor in medicine. Since it seemed to behave a little like ordinary magnetism, he called the life force "animal magnetism" and concluded that it filled the entire cosmos and could be stored, transmitted, and used either to heal or to harm. He worked out a series of protocols for collecting it and applying it to patients, using tubs of water as well as his own body and that of his students, and accomplished impressive cures. More orthodox scientists, incensed by these heresies, soon made Vienna too hot for him, and Mesmer relocated to Paris, where he achieved fame and fortune but became the focus of even more controversy. Embittered by the attacks on his reputation and his discoveries, he retired to Switzerland in old age and died there in 1815.

After his death, Mesmer's legacy was reworked in several different ways. The one that most people know about was launched in 1842 by Scottish physician James Braid. This was a straightforward matter

---

[2] John McClenon's *Deviant Science* is a good sociological study of the ways in which taboos of this kind are enforced. See McClenon 1984.

of taking some of Mesmer's practices out of context, discarding his theory, renaming the resulting watered-down system "hypnotism," and marketing it under that new label. Other researchers explored the more controversial aspects of Mesmer's work, but they were exiled to the fringes as he was, and accordingly received much less attention from the general public.

Two of these offshoots are of special importance in our inquiry. The first was siderism, which was developed by the brilliant German scientist Johann Wilhelm Ritter, the discoverer of ultraviolet light and the inventor of electroplating. Siderism (from the Latin word *siderus*, "star, celestial object") took its starting point from Mesmer's doctoral dissertation, which explored the possibility that movements of the sun, moon, and planets relative to earth might affect the movements of animal magnetism in the cosmos. Ritter's early death and the vicious reaction of the scientific mainstream to anything that could be seen as a justification for astrology quickly drove siderism to the cultural fringes.

The same fate awaited tellurism, another system of thought and practice based on Mesmer's original work. This was the creation of Dietrich Georg von Kieser, a German physician and university professor, and came to public notice by way of one of Kieser's many books, *System des Tellurismus oder thierischen Magnetismus* (*System of Tellurism or Animal Magnetism*), published in 1826. Tellurism (from the Latin word *tellus*, "Earth") worked with currents of the life force moving in and around the Earth. It identified the magnetic poles and the magnetic field of the planet as sources of animal magnetism and tracked the movements of the life force through the ground in patterns that are sometimes suggestive of the Chinese art of *feng shui*. While it was chased out of the mainstream along with the rest of Mesmer's legacy, it found a welcome in a variety of fringe traditions in the German- and English-speaking countries after Kieser's time.

One measure of the spread of tellurism in the cultural underground is a series of articles that appeared in 1835 and 1836 in *The Shepherd*, an eclectic English periodical that catered to the alternative culture of the time. The articles were titled "Letters on Tellurism, Commonly Called Animal Magnetism." They appeared under yet another pseudonym, "the Alpine Philosopher." The author was Gioacchino de Prati, an Italian writer and Mesmerist then living in England as a political exile. They present a cosmology in which two great currents, a solar current and a telluric (terrestrial) current, generate life by their ebb and flow.

"The Alpine Philosopher" apparently knew nothing of Abby Judson's exercise, but the text of her booklet makes it clear that she was working in the same tradition, drawing on the same ideas. Judson saw magnetism—the term "animal" dropped out of use in alternative culture in the English-speaking countries by the second half of the nineteenth century—as a force that emanated from the north pole of the Earth and flowed southward. It could be absorbed by the practitioner and used in various ways, and her exercises were among the ways to draw on the life force of the planet and put it to practical use. De Prati's approach uses different means of tapping into the life force but the underlying theory is the same.

ဢ

Behind Judson's borrowing of concepts from tellurism was the wholesale adoption of Mesmer's ideas by the Spiritualist movement of the nineteenth century. The most influential figure in the early decades of American Spiritualism, the writer and trance medium Andrew Jackson Davis, began his career after being put into trance by a traveling Mesmerist, and his voluminous books on the spirit world drew heavily on Mesmerist ideas. The entire concept of entering into trance in order to channel the voices of the dead came to the Spiritualist movement from Mesmerists, who experimented with the psychic perceptions of people in trance decades before Spiritualism emerged.

Abby Judson was one of many Spiritualists who made use of the resulting fusion of ideas. Spiritualism and the broader American occult community, however, interpenetrated in a galaxy of ways all through the nineteenth century, and Mesmerist terminology was borrowed just as enthusiastically by occultists as by Spiritualists. Read volumes on occultism published in the United States during the half century or so before the publication of *The Eye of Revelation* and it's hard to miss finding talk about magnetism, trance states, and interactions between living human beings and a dizzying range of disembodied entities. The biography of Harry J. Gardener is among other things a testimony to the resulting overlap: as mentioned in Chapter One, he began his occult studies by studying Spiritualism alongside his father and proceeded from there to take up the distinctive form of occultism that helped shape *The Eye of Revelation*.

It was by way of these linkages that the exercise Abby Judson learned from her teacher, or some other exercise very close to it, seems to have found its way into one of the circles of occultists who worked with the exercises that became the Five Rites. As Charles B. Roth's version of the exercises in *Hindu Secrets* demonstrates, there were certainly people working with the same set of exercises who either never encountered Judson's practice or saw no point in including it. Somewhere along the line, however, it appears that a practice closely related to Judson's exercises found its way to the version of the exercises that reached Peter Kelder, and became the First Rite.

The current of thought that passed from Mesmer to Judson and then to *The Eye of Revelation* left other traces in Kelder's booklet. The seven vortices in the body that play a central role in Kelder's version of the exercises, though not in Roth's, are described as "magnetic centers" as well as "psychic vortexes," for example; the magnetism that Kelder has in mind is clearly not the sort that will attract bits of iron! More significant is the way that Kelder's book stresses the direction of rotation in the First Rite. This must always be clockwise. Why? Kelder does not say. Judson's booklet provides the missing detail.

According to her explanation, clockwise rotation draws in magnetism, while counterclockwise rotation "throws off the currents." Her exercise thus starts with a dispersing movement to cleanse the body of unwanted animal magnetism and then uses a larger number of clockwise rotations to recharge the body with the life force. The First Rite is simpler in conception and practice but it draws on the same structure of ideas. The first task of the practitioner of the Five Rites, in this way of thinking, is to charge the body with extra magnetism. The later Rites then work with it so that the seven vortices are filled with the life force and spin at their proper speed.

Kelder was apparently unaware of this dimension of the First Rite, or at least he did not mention it in his booklet. Since Judson's exercise had been published decades earlier with a full explanation of its energetic work, it is unlikely that Kelder considered the subject too secret to write about in a booklet for sale to the public. This suggests that the First Rite had been added to the other four before Kelder received it, though it also suggests that the philosophy underling the Five Rites may not have been fully understood by those who put it into print.

Such lapses are far from uncommon in the history of occultism. It is sometimes possible, however, to spot hints and clues in published sources that allow the underlying philosophy and context of a practice to be reconstructed. Fortunately, the Five Rites have several such clues. One of them, so simple as to pass unnoticed, is the instruction in *The Eye of Revelation* and *Hindu Secrets* to wash daily in cool or tepid water. It is to this that we now turn.

CHAPTER 4

The Waters

Most people in industrial societies nowadays think of bathing as an ordinary chore of daily life, with little connection to health and less connection to spirituality. In the days before cheap energy and petrochemicals made hot water and soap easily accessible throughout the industrial world, however, bathing was a more significant event, and its subtler dimensions were better understood. To this day, orthodox Jews treat the *mikveh* or ritual bathing facility as an essential part of their religious lives, devout Hindus regard a pilgrimage to bathe in the sacred waters of the Ganges as the spiritual high point of an entire incarnation, and people around the world use water to purify themselves ceremonially before setting foot inside churches, mosques, temples, and shrines.

From the point of view of the occult traditions of the West, all this makes perfect sense. Water is a vehicle for the life force we discussed in the previous chapter.[1] It can absorb, store, and transmit a wide range of subtle influences. (That was why Mesmer used tubs of water as reservoirs of animal magnetism.) Broadly speaking, there are two principal uses for water in occult practice: it can be used to bring some

---

[1] See, among many other sources, Ramacharaka 1908, pp. 6–10.

desired influence to a person or object that lacks it, or it can be used to take away an unwanted influence from a person or object burdened with it.

The first of these applications is the principle behind holy water. When water is blessed by a holy person, or otherwise passed through some process that charges it with beneficent influences, it holds onto those influences and can transmit them to anything that comes into contact with the water. The second application, in turn, is the principle behind bathing as a means of spiritual purification, because washing in water can take away metaphysical impurities just as effectively as their physical equivalents. Occult theory has it that the world we live in is just as full of magnetic impurities as it is of physical dirt, and both need to be washed off.

Both these effects were known in the occult counterculture of the early twentieth century. Occultists at the time had another reason to be interested in the properties of water, however. Then as now, there was a substantial overlap between occultism and alternative health-care modalities, and one of the nineteenth century's most widely used forms of alternative health care was still popular during the period when the Five Rites were taking shape. This was hydropathy, or as it was also called, the water cure.

Most forms of alternative health care have colorful origin stories, and hydropathy is better than most. Though people have been using hot, tepid, and cold baths for healing purposes since the dawn of history, the modern movement began with a young Austrian farmer named Vincenz Priessnitz. As a boy, Preissnitz witnessed a wounded deer bathing in a pond near his home; the deer returned to the pond day after day, until it was completely healed of its wounds. Later, as a teenager, he had a farm cart run over him, breaking several of his ribs. When the local doctor told him that the ribs would never heal, Priessnitz thought of the deer. By using frequent cold wet bandages and drinking large quantities of water, he cured the broken ribs in a year.

As an adult, Preissnitz opened a clinic where patients were treated with cold water baths and bandages and given large quantities of fresh water to drink. This regimen, combined with plain healthy meals and plenty of gentle exercises, such as long walks in the countryside, brought about many cures. In response, hydropathy centers opened in countries all over the Western world. Most of these used some variant of

Preissnitz's original system, emphasizing large amounts of cold water to a degree that very often shocked the system of the patient.

A less rigorous approach to hydropathy came in with Preissnitz's most influential successor, Father Sebastian Kneipp, a Bavarian priest who ended up devoting his life to the water cure. He retained the use of cold water baths for those strong enough to benefit from them and even put snow into the water tank in winter, but he was also capable of a gentler approach: "To beginners in the water-cure, to weak persons, especially very young or very old ones, to sick people who are afraid of a cold, to such as have not much warmth in their blood, whose blood is poor, or who are nervous, I gladly allow, especially in winter-time, a warm room for their baths and showers (65 degrees) for the beginning, and lukewarm water for every application."[2]

Over the course of the nineteenth century, the water cure accordingly spun off two competing schools of hydropathy, the proponents of which bickered with one another in much the same way as the proponents of gymnastics and calisthenics or those of hatha yoga and *Surya Namaskar* did. (Surprisingly enough, I have been unable to find evidence for similar squabbles between practitioners of siderism and tellurism.) On one side was the cold water system, which was associated with the physical culture movement, the great nineteenth- and early twentieth century push for healthy exercise and natural living. The cold water system appealed mostly to men and to the already healthy who wanted to become more fit than they already were.

On the other side was the warm water system, which was especially popular among women and the genuinely unwell. Its practitioners condemned the cold water system as being nearly as lethal as other popular Victorian forms of medical practice: "The signal neglect to apply external heat to organs deficient in vitality is the grand defect of all allopathic or homoeopathic practice, and the cause of the death of innumerable human beings," wrote Caroline Anne Smedley, a popular author of the warm water school, and went on: "Vital heat is life; deficiency of it weakness and disease; absence of it death."[3]

The two schools had different understandings of the way that water can be used to heal. The cold water approach focused on shocking the system in order to throw the metabolism into high gear and saw

[2] Kneipp 1896, p. 16.
[3] Smedley 1878., p. 1.

closing the pores of the skin as a benefit, arguing that disease organisms could enter the body through open pores. The warm water approach argued instead that fostering warmth in the internal organs was essential and saw opening the skin pores as a benefit, arguing that wastes could be expelled from the body through the pores. Gentle exercise played a significant role in some versions of the warm water system. Colonel Bradford's warning in *The Eye of Revelation* came straight from this approach: "You must never take a shower, tub, or wet towel bath which is cold enough to chill you even slightly internally. If you do, you will have undone all the good you have gained from performing the Five Rites."

Most authorities nowadays like to dismiss hydropathy as quack medicine, though of course that same label gets used reliably for any healing modality that doesn't bring in profits for the medical and pharmaceutical industries. To judge by contemporary sources, it seems to have helped a great many people with chronic conditions improve their health. How much of that had to do with healthy eating, gentle exercise, and adequate hydration is admittedly hard to answer from the evidence at hand, but including water baths in the system of the Five Rites was a way to align the exercises with what was still a widely accepted form of alternative healing in 1939.

☙

The literature of hydropathy allows very precise lines to be drawn between the contending schools of practice discussed above. According to Dr. R.T. Trall's *Hydropathic Encyclopedia*, water counted as "cold" from 40° to 55°F, as "cool" from 55° to 65°F, and as "tepid" from 72° to 85°F. (Between cool and tepid in Trall's system was another category, "temperate.") From 85°F to normal body temperature was "warm," and above that was "hot." The creators and promulgators of the Five Rites, by specifying cool or tepid baths, thus clearly intended to strike a middle ground between the cold water and warm water schools.

That same approach was a commonplace of occult teachings from the same period. One classic example was yet another booklet by the prolific William Walker Atkinson, writing this time as Yogi Ramacharaka. The instructions in *The Hindu-Yogi System of Practical Water Cure* inevitably had nothing to do with Hindu teachings or yoga practices. Like most of Atkinson's "Yoga" works, they came straight out of European alternative culture, with a thin frosting of Oriental imagery and rhetoric spread over the top. Here as elsewhere, Atkinson's great value to a modern researcher is his sheer lack of originality; the teachings he presents are an excellent guide to the common occult traditions and practices of his day.

Atkinson's discussion of the water cure thus shows a good practical knowledge of the standard hydropathy literature of his time and takes a middle line among the contending parties. He recommended cold baths for those whose bodies were strong enough to benefit from them, but what he meant by a cold bath was a little more lenient than Vincenz Preissnitz or Father Kneipp had in mind: "In fact, we may say that any bath below blood-heat (98 degrees) may be considered a Cold Bath, the degree of coolness corresponding to the vitality of the bather—the more vital, the colder the water, down to a limit which ordinary sanity will enforce."[4]

While Atkinson discusses the benefits of cold baths, hot baths, and most of the other standard elements of the water cure, his recommendation for daily practice is the same one that appears in Kelder's and Roth's booklets. His "Daily Cleansing Bath" used lukewarm water, "neither so cold as to chill one, nor so hot as to produce the feeling of great heat."[5] This is close enough to the advice in *The Eye of Revelation* and *Hindu Secrets* that the possibility of direct borrowing should again be taken into account. Since the Five Rites themselves may be descended from Exercise XI in Atkinson's *Hatha Yoga*, as we have seen, and since Atkinson's writings were extraordinarily influential in American occultism during the years when the Five Rites emerged, some such connection is more likely than not.

All this casts a useful light on *The Eye of Revelation* and *Hindu Secrets*. Both books make it clear that the Five Rites (or four *dands*) are not primarily intended for those who are already in robust health. In fact, Peter Kelder specifically distances his system from the physical culture movement.[6] He and Charles B. Roth both aimed their pamphlets at readers who were in ordinary health at best and were not prepared to invest the time and effort required by the physical culture teachers of the time. Their stated goal was to provide a simple set of exercises, taking only a few minutes a day, which could maintain the practitioner in good health into advanced old age. The very simple form of the water

---

[4] Ramacharaka 1908, p. 94.
[5] Ramacharaka 1908, p. 89.
[6] See below, p. xx.

cure included in both books, a lukewarm bath each day, was another expression of that same approach: a means of health that was less strenuous than physical culture but was still quite effective.

It is worth remembering, though, that the Five Rites were not simply physical exercises. They always had a metaphysical dimension, as we will see in the chapters ahead. The use of tepid or cool water baths may also have had a dimension beyond that of ordinary physical health. The life force, the secret power behind Abby Judson's exercise and the First Rite, is likely to be involved here as well.

A scrap of lore widespread in occult circles from the late nineteenth century on measures the capacity of water to hold animal magnetism by its temperature. According to this teaching, water reaches its maximum capacity to absorb magnetism at 39°F and becomes completely unable to absorb magnetism at 97°–99°F—that is, at normal body temperature. Warm water may be suitable for providing vital heat, as Caroline Anne Smedley thought, but it will not take away the magnetic impurities that clutter up our environments. Cold water does the best possible job of removing these impurities, but may be too much of a shock to the system for regular use by the elderly, ailing, or sensitive. Tepid or cool water strikes a workable balance between these two extremes.

It has to be said that there is no explicit evidence anywhere in *The Eye of Revelation* to suggest an occult dimension to the tepid water baths Kelder suggests. As so often, it is necessary to proceed by inference from the scraps of knowledge that can be gathered. In the case of the seven vortices, the theme of the next chapter, there is much less uncertainty, since the only other places I know of where these centers are discussed include one of the core works of classic American occultism and a set of correspondence lessons offered by an influential American occult order.

CHAPTER 5

The Vortices

The seven vortices that feature in *The Eye of Revelation* are among the most distinctive aspects of Peter Kelder's teachings. They are all but unique in the world's occult, spiritual, and esoteric traditions. Systems of energy centers in the body are of course found all over the world. The seven chakras of Hindu tradition, located in the spine and brain, are one set that most people in the Western world know about these days. Many other sets of energy centers are described in the world's spiritual writings and teachings, to be sure, but the seven vortices Peter Kelder discussed are to be found only in a few distinctive sources.

The vortices will play a sufficiently important role in the discussion ahead that it's worth taking a moment to describe them in detail here. They are located at certain specific points in the physical body, as listed below, and are centers of magnetism—that is to say, the life force. Their strength, and the vitality of the person to whom they belong, can be gauged by the speed and strength of their rotation: the faster they rotate, the better.

Vortex A, to use Kelder's label for it, is located inside the forehead. Vortex B is in the back of the brain. Vortex C is in the region of the throat, just inward from the little notch between the collarbones at the base of

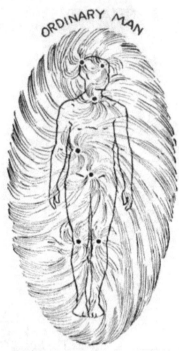

CURRENTS IN THE DESIRE BODY

the neck in front. Vortex D is on the right side of the torso above the waistline, in the area of the liver, roughly halfway between the front and back surface of the trunk. Vortex E is just above and inward from the base of the penis or clitoris, and vortices F and G are inside the knee joints. Kelder also notes that there is an important connection between the throat center C and the genital center E—a point that will be worth keeping in mind as we proceed.

Unusual as they are, these centers can be found well documented in a very small number of sources dating from well before 1939. When *The Eye of Revelation* first saw print, in fact, it is a safe bet that most of the occult bookshops that carried it also sold *The Rosicrucian Cosmo-Conception* by Max Heindel, one of the most widely read American occult manuals of the time. Nowadays, though Heindel's volume remains in print, you have to look a little harder to find copies for sale, and apparently, very few of the people who practice the Five Rites at present have ever encountered it.

This is unfortunate. Had they turned the pages of *The Rosicrucian Cosmo-Conception*, they would have found good clear illustrations of the same seven vortices that Kelder included in his booklet. In my copy of Heindel's book, they are between pages 66 and 67, three black and white plates labeled "Currents in the Desire Body," showing the human aura with the seven whirling vortices exactly where *The Eye of Revelation* put them. The text of Heindel's book, furthermore, uses the term "vortices" for these centers of subtle energy and stresses that they should rotate in a clockwise direction. It also discusses at some length the subtle linkages between the genitals and the throat center.

The Rosicrucian Cosmo-Conception was originally published in 1909. It is the primary textbook of the Rosicrucian Fellowship, the organization founded by Max Heindel to pass on his esoteric teachings. The Fellowship exists today and is still headquartered in Oceanside, California, as mentioned back in Chapter One. It describes itself as an association of Christian mystics offering training to aspirants through correspondence courses in astrology and occult philosophy with a Christian slant. Members are encouraged to take up celibacy and vegetarian diets and practice spiritual exercises every morning and evening.

These exercises are intended to develop the same seven vortices that are described in *The Eye of Revelation*. The Fellowship's exercises are nothing like the Five Rites, and they are not meant to grant longevity and vitality. Their purpose is the development of the hidden powers of the human soul—in particular, the development of the ability to see the spiritual worlds directly and replace speculations about the Unseen with direct personal knowledge. One traditional way to talk about this ability is to call it the opening of the Eye of Revelation.

ଓଃ

There is a long and fascinating backstory to *The Rosicrucian Cosmo-Conception* and the teachings that it contains. Max Heindel, the founder of the Rosicrucian Fellowship, was another of the many pseudonymous figures in our story. His name was originally Carl Grashof. He was Danish by birth, worked as a ship's engineer, and became fluent in English while studying for his trade in Edinburgh. He also had a lifelong interest in Christian occultism. That interest brought him into contact with some of the most influential occultists of his time and eventually sent him to the United States and his destiny as a spiritual teacher.

According to Heindel's own account, it was while he was in Europe in 1906 that he made contact with a senior occultist he called simply the Elder Brother. This person, according to Heindel's account, was a member of the secret order of Rosicrucians and assigned him the task of bringing the Rosicrucian teachings to America.

The Rosicrucians, the brothers of the Rose Cross, play a fascinating role in the history of Western occultism. The entire Rosicrucian phenomenon started as an unusually successful college prank. A group of students at the University of Tübingen in Germany sometime around 1609 worked up a manifesto, the *Fama Fraternitatis* ("News of the Fraternity"), proclaiming the existence of a secret society of German adepts—the Rosicrucians, or Brothers of the Rose Cross—founded by a mysterious adept called C.R.C., who knew everything worth knowing about everything. The pamphlet invited all and sundry to apply for membership by writing letters and publishing them in the pamphlet press, the seventeenth century equivalent of Facebook. This narrative was printed in 1614 in the same pamphlet as the German translation of a raucous Italian satire titled *General Reformation of the Whole Wide World*, in which Apollo calls together a convention of wise men to solve the problems of the world, listens to their harebrained schemes, and then imposes price controls on cabbages, upon which everyone goes home rejoicing. It's clear from context that the whole thing was intended as a joke, the sort of thing that earned the *Harvard Lampoon* its reputation in a later century.

Germany in the early seventeenth century was a seething cauldron of religious and political passions teetering on the verge of civil war. In such an environment, even the most harmless sort of humor can spin out of control. That was what happened with the *Fama Fraternitatis*. No one seems to have recognized it as a satire. People all over Europe responded to its publication with frantic attempts to find the mysterious brotherhood, either to join it or to burn its members at the stake. Two other publications appeared, the *Confessio Fraternitatis* and the *Alchemical Wedding of Christian Rosycross*, throwing more fuel on an already blazing fire. By the time the Thirty Years War broke out in 1618, a great many people were convinced of the existence of the Rosicrucian Brotherhood.

Once the fighting finally wound up in 1648 and Germany began to recover from the long ordeal, Rosicrucian societies began to appear in a handful of European countries and expanded from that beginning over the years that followed. By the time Max Heindel went looking for Rosicrucians in Europe, accordingly, Rosicrucian lodges had been active in Germany and several other European countries for at least two and a half centuries. Rosicrucianism had become one of the established flavors of Western occult study and practice, with lodges sponsored by dozens of competing Rosicrucian orders on every continent but Antarctica.

Among the most influential figures in European Rosicrucian circles at the time of Heindel's visit was the Christian mystic Alois Mailander, who lived in seclusion near Darmstadt in southern Germany. Mailander was a nearly illiterate weaver who taught and practiced a system of Christian mysticism based on the teachings of two earlier Christian mystics, Jacob Boehme and J.B. Kerning. Though he is rarely remembered today, Mailander's personal qualities and his mastery of abstruse spiritual philosophy attracted attention from many central European occultists at the time, and the Theosophical lodges in Vienna and Prague were particularly interested in his teachings.

In 1889, while their interest in Mailander was at its peak, the Vienna Theosophists welcomed a new member named Rudolf Steiner, a young Austrian intellectual who was also a rising star in the world of mainstream scholarship. The following year, Steiner would be asked to edit the scientific works of Goethe for a new standard edition, and a few years after that he would shock the European intellectual scene by coming out publicly as an occultist. In later years, Steiner credited a teacher he called simply "M" for much of his inspiration. Several recent researchers have shown that the mysterious "M" was almost certainly Mailander. Many of Mailander's students called him "the Elder Brother," furthermore, and it has been argued that Mailander was the Elder Brother that Max Heindel met during his travels in Europe. Certainly, Heindel's teachings, with their devout if quirky Christian piety, seem closely akin to what is known about the teachings Mailander communicated to his students.

గ్ర

Yet there may have been more involved in Heindel's last trip to Europe than this suggests. A story that has been in circulation for years now among European Rosicrucians and students of Rudolf Steiner casts a fascinating light on Heindel's connection with Steiner and the events behind the foundation of the Rosicrucian Fellowship. In the nature of such things, it is impossible to know just how accurate an account of events it offers, but it is worth considering.

Here is the story.[1] In 1906, as he became increasingly active in occult circles, Rudolf Steiner founded what he hoped would become the most important occult order in Europe, the Mystica Aeterna (Eternal Mystic). To spread the teachings of the Mystica Aeterna, Steiner set out to recruit an Inner Circle of twelve senior occultists, one from each of twelve European countries. Edouard Schuré, a famous French author of occult books, was the member for France; Giovanni Colazza, a leading Italian occultist, represented Italy; Andrei Belyi from Russia, Gustav Meyrink from Austria, and Alexander von Bernus from Germany are also said to have belonged to the Inner Circle. Max Heindel was another member, and Steiner intended him as the member for Denmark.

At least in theory, this was not simply a matter of politics within the occult community. It had a deeper spiritual dimension. Steiner believed that he was called to lead a series of powerful rituals, which he called "Mystery Dramas," that would literally transform the world. He wanted to unite all occult traditions under the banner of the Mystica Aeterna in order to further the cause of the great transformation. The members of the Inner Circle were meant to assist at the last of those rituals, which would bring the Christ Spirit into manifestation and usher in a new age of the world. An extraordinary wooden building, the Goetheanum, was constructed in Dornach, Switzerland as a setting for these rites.

The members of the Inner Circle received a set of Rosicrucian teachings from Steiner and were expected to publish these in their own languages. Schuré released the teachings in France under the title *Évolution Divine* (*Divine Evolution*), and Steiner prepared them for publication in German. For reasons of his own, however, Heindel refused to take the role that Steiner had assigned him. Instead, he left Europe for the United States, settling first in Seattle and then in Oceanside, California, and published the teachings in English instead. This was in direct contradiction with Steiner's intentions, for Steiner felt that his Rosicrucian teachings needed to be established in Europe before they could be conveyed to the New World.

Heindel insisted that he had been tasked by his Rosicrucian teacher, the Elder Brother, to communicate the teachings to the New World. His departure threw Steiner's plans into disarray. In 1914, with only

---

[1] The version I have given here is based primarily on Cosmic Convergence Research Group (2017).

four of the projected seven Mystery Dramas written, Steiner dissolved the Mystica Aeterna. In 1922, after the first version of the Goetheanum was burnt to the ground by an arsonist, Steiner rebuilt the Goetheanum to a different design and made it from concrete instead of wood. At the same time, he dropped most of his connections with the European occult scene and shelved his hopes of transforming the world.

Meanwhile, Heindel had established his own school at Oceanside, published the teachings in *The Rosicrucian Cosmo-Conception*, and attracted a steady stream of students. The first edition of *The Rosicrucian Cosmo-Conception* was dedicated to Rudolf Steiner, though Heindel removed the dedication in later editions after Steiner denounced him in 1913. Neither Heindel nor Steiner ever discussed publicly the events that led to their going separate ways.

It is worth noting, however, that Heindel's teachings stayed strictly away from grandiose visions of the kind that motivated Steiner's founding of the Mystica Aeterna and focused instead on the far more pragmatic mission of teaching Rosicrucian philosophy, astrology, and spiritual healing to students in America and other countries. It may simply be that Steiner's sense of his own exalted spiritual importance and his habit of claiming that everything that happened to him reflected vast happenings in the spiritual world were ultimately too much for Heindel to take, and Heindel decided to distance himself from Steiner for this reason.

The relevance of all this to our story is simply that it hints at some of Heindel's connections in the European Rosicrucian scene. When he left Europe for the United States, Heindel brought with him an extensive body of teachings, including much of the raw material that went into *The Rosicrucian Cosmo-Conception* and at least some of the rituals of the Aeterna Mystica. What else he might have brought with him is an open question, but as we will see in a later chapter, the seven vortices were almost certainly among the teachings he learned in Europe.

ᴄᴈ

The Rosicrucian Fellowship was not the only American Rosicrucian group that knew about the seven vortices. In 1908, while Max Heindel was working on the final proofs for *The Rosicrucian Cosmo-Conception*, a young Freemason named George Winslow Plummer was initiated into the Rosicrucian tradition by an Elder Brother of his own. Sylvester Gould, the initiator in question, was a longtime Freemason who had received his own Rosicrucian initiation sometime in the middle years of the nineteenth century and had extensive contacts in the European occult scene. He had been planning for some time to launch a Rosicrucian order in the United States. The two men promptly drew up plans for such an order. In 1909, however, Gould unexpectedly died, and Plummer took on the project by himself. The Societas Rosicruciana in America (SRIA) was duly organized in 1912 with Plummer as its head.

Following the same trajectory as Heindel's organization, and many other occult orders of the same period, the SRIA promptly started publishing books of Rosicrucian philosophy and practice written by Plummer. There was also an extensive series of correspondence lessons, also written by Plummer, which were made available to members of the order. The most important of the books, *Rosicrucian Fundamentals*, appeared in 1920, but *Rosicrucian Symbology* (1916) and *Rosicrucian Manual* (1923) are also significant guides to the SRIA's teachings. Plummer was somewhat more closemouthed about the inner dimensions of his teachings than Heindel, however, and the seven vortices do not appear in any of the books just cited.

On the other hand, they can be found in a diagram included with an undated lecture of Plummer's, titled "Those Alchemists—Our Glands," which can be found on the internet in many places as of this writing. These same vortices also play a significant role in the private lessons issued by the SRIA during Plummer's lifetime. There is one odd variation in Plummer's system: where Kelder and Heindel place the vortex in the middle of the trunk on the right side and associate it with the liver, Plummer places it on the left side and associates it with the spleen. As we will see, this has its own lesson to teach.

As in Heindel's book, the energy centers listed in Plummer's lecture and lessons are called vortices, and the point is stressed that they should always turn in a clockwise direction. Plummer's lessons also explain at some length that the psychic centers or vortices in the throat and genitals are linked and form the positive and negative poles of the human aura.[2]

Where Plummer got his information about the vortices is a fascinating question that cannot yet be answered on the basis of the available evidence. He was unquestionably familiar with Heindel's work, as he cites *The Rosicrucian Cosmo-Conception* repeatedly in the pages of

---

[2] Spiritual Alchemy course lesson 2, pp. 1–3.

Rosicrucian Fundamentals, and he could have learned about the vortices from that source. He also cites Steiner's work in the same book. Equally, however, he had a range of other contacts in the occult community of his time, and his teacher Sylvester Gould had an even broader range of connections.

There is at least one detail in Plummer's writings that suggests some source of knowledge about the vortices independent of Heindel. He mentions in one of his advanced lessons that concentration on the vortices was an important part of training in "many occult schools and brotherhoods." The two centers in the knees, he notes, were the usual initial point at which this part of the work of spiritual alchemy began.[3]

Plummer himself did not favor this approach and argued instead that practitioners should concentrate on the solar plexus. Thus it's unlikely that he invented the practice of concentrating on the knee centers and then marketed it as an ancient secret teaching—a habit by no means rare in occult circles. I have found no trace of either of these details anywhere in Heindel's writings. The most likely explanation for this is that Plummer had some independent source for his knowledge of the vortices and their use in occult training.

The training he passed on to his students had some close parallels to Heindel's system and some notable differences. It's possible to be precise about these points, because both men took what was then an unusual step and published their orders' introductory methods of practice in books available to the general public—Heindel in *The Rosicrucian Cosmo-Conception* and Plummer in *Rosicrucian Manual*.[4] Both taught their students to spend a few minutes on going to bed each night recalling everything that had happened during the day, a classic occult practice dating to ancient Greek times; both taught their students to spend a few minutes on waking up each morning concentrating on a spiritual ideal; and both taught the use of the Lord's Prayer as a daily spiritual practice.

Heindel insisted on a vegetarian diet and a vow of chastity, however, while Plummer explicitly denied that either of these were worth taking up as general rules. Plummer's system recommends a diet high in fruits and vegetables, but the only meats that are forbidden are pork and veal, and he insisted that sexual activity was entirely up to the choice of the practitioner. Plummer also instructed his students to perform a breathing

---

[3] Spiritual Alchemy course lesson 4, p. 6.
[4] Heindel 1909, pp. 430–97 and 601–06; Plummer 1923, pp. 35–7.

exercise every morning and to wash their bodies daily in tepid water, while Heindel mentioned neither of these in his public writings.

Another curious difference between the Rosicrucian teachings of Heindel and Plummer has to do with another set of five centers subsidiary to the seven vortices. Both men included references to such a secondary set in their instructional writings, but they disagreed about what the secondary set was. In Heindel's teachings, the five additional centers are the palms of both hands, the soles of both feet, and the outer surface of the head and face; these were the parts of the body of Jesus that were wounded at his crucifixion, the hands and feet by nails and the head and face by the crown of thorns. Heindel saw these as the places where the physical body and the body of life force were most closely bound together, and where that binding had to be loosened in order to permit the soul to travel out of the body.[5]

To Plummer, by contrast, the five additional centers were the two breasts, the solar plexus, the heart, and the base of the spine.[6] It seems clear, in other words, that one or both men received a set of teachings that were at least partly incomplete; the material seems to have mentioned that there were five additional centers, but what those centers might be was not explained, and some combination of study and clairvoyance had to be used to fill in the gaps. (For whatever it may be worth, my own experiments suggest that Heindel was correct, but more research needs to be done to confirm this.)

One thing that Heindel and Plummer unquestionably shared, however, was a sense of the purpose of the exercises they taught. Both saw the point of occult training as the development of the ability to experience the spiritual worlds directly. The chapter in *The Rosicrucian Cosmo-Conception* on spiritual practice is titled "The Method of Acquiring First-Hand Knowledge," while the explicitly defined purpose of Plummer's lessons on spiritual alchemy is the awakening of clairvoyant abilities. This same approach, it is worth noting, pervades the writings of Rudolf Steiner, who (especially in his early writings) presented the goal of his training as the attainment of seership.[7] Another way to describe the same process, of course, is the opening of the Eye of Revelation.

---

[5] Heindel 1950, p. 149.
[6] Spiritual Alchemy course lesson 1, p. 3.
[7] See, for example, Steiner 1908.

CHAPTER 6

The Glands

Important as they are, the seven vortices share space in the tradition we are discussing with another set of centers, more material in nature. These are the endocrine glands or, as they were often called in the early twentieth century, the ductless glands. Charles B. Roth's *Hindu Secrets of Vitality and Rejuvenation*, as we have seen, interprets its exercises as ways to stimulate the endocrine glands instead of the seven vortices. This isn't a mistake or a distortion. The vortices and the glands are both involved in the system that gave rise to the Five Rites.

The endocrine glands are a set of organs, most of them small, scattered through the head and trunk of the human body. Their function is to produce hormones, most of which are released directly into the bloodstream. These glands include the hypothalamus and the pituitary and pineal glands, on the underside of the brain; the thyroid, which wraps around the windpipe, and the parathyroid glands, which are directly behind the thyroid; the thymus, in the upper chest; the pancreas, located below and behind the stomach; the adrenal glands, located on top of both kidneys; the ovaries and testes, connected to the female and male genitals respectively; and an assortment of little clusters of cells located all through the vital organs and the skin, which make their own contributions to the intricate symphony of hormones in the blood. (The coccygeal glomus, a supposedly vestigial gland at the base of the spine, may also belong with the endocrine organs, though current Western medicine knows nothing about any hormones it may secrete.) Some writers in Harry Gardener's time also considered the spleen and the liver to be endocrine organs because of their importance in the hormonal system.

The role of the endocrine system in health and disease was unsuspected by Western medical researchers until 1921. That was when Canadian researchers discovered that insulin produced by the pancreas was essential to the body to maintain blood sugar balance. Further discoveries followed promptly, revealing more of the endocrine system's functions in the body, and headlines splashed the news all over the news media of the time. As a result, the endocrine glands received a great deal of public interest all through the 1920s and 1930s. It's indicative that in India, where those same years saw hatha yoga complete much of its twentieth century transition from spiritual discipline to health exercise, the headlines caught the eye of yoga researcher and teacher Swami Kuvalayananda (J.G. Gune). From the 1920s on, Kuvalayananda's writings publicized hatha yoga as a way to stimulate the endocrine glands into activity, with a range of health benefits.[1]

The same ideas inevitably found their way into Western occultism as well. The two American Rosicrucian orders we have been discussing were particularly quick to explore possible linkages between their teachings and the new discoveries about endocrine function. George Winslow Plummer's article "Those Alchemists—Our Glands" cited in the previous chapter is a revealing example. It presents an overview of the endocrine system as understood by scientists at the time and then goes in an unexpected direction:

> [I]n the alchemy of the human body all the legitimate and traditional processes of alchemy are developed by the glands in the exercise of their several and individual functions. Fermentatio, Putrefactio, Sublimatio, Condensatio, Calcinatio,[2] etc., are active in the exact formulae prescribed by the ancient writers, and the distilled product veils a secret Principle, unknown even to the foremost researchers in glandular activity, that functions in the development and

---

[1] Goldberg 2016, pp. 86–7.
[2] These are among the phases of the alchemical process in traditional alchemical writings.

manifestation of human traits we have hitherto been led to accept as works of the Spirit that is in Man. Perhaps we are tracing that spirit in Man to its very lair. Perhaps the endocrine glands will prove to be the threshold of the entrance from the Seen to the Unseen.[3]

Plummer is here using the language of alchemy, one of the occult traditions long associated with the Rosicrucian movement. Like many Rosicrucian writers—and also, of course, other scholars such as the psychologist Carl Jung—he held that the laboratory jargon of alchemy was meant to conceal something unrelated to physical glassware and metallic gold. What he is suggesting in this passage, and elsewhere in his writings, is that the true alchemical vessel is the human body, and the materials of alchemy are the secretions of the endocrine glands.

CB

The 1936 pamphlet *Astrology and the Ductless Glands*, a more lengthy examination of the glands written by Max Heindel's widow Augusta Foss Heindel, is even more revealing in its own way. It assigned planets to those of the endocrine glands the Rosicrucian Fellowship teachings were willing to discuss—the pineal gland was associated with Neptune, the pituitary gland with Uranus, the thyroid with Mercury, the thymus with Venus, and the adrenals with Jupiter. The pituitary and pineal glands get the lion's share of the discussion, as they usually do in Rosicrucian literature (and especially in the writings of the Rosicrucian Fellowship). Rejuvenation is mentioned in the pamphlet, but only so that the author can insist primly that diet and pure thinking are the only true Fountain of Youth.[4]

The art of noticing what is not being said is essential in the study of occult traditions, and Augusta Heindel's booklet needs to be read with this in mind. Nowhere does she mention Mars or Saturn, nor are the testes and ovaries referenced at all. The system of seven vortices found in *The Rosicrucian Cosmo-Conception* has been replaced by seven endocrine glands at waist level or above. Yet it's a simple matter to work back from Augusta Heindel's list to the planetary correspondences of the seven vortices.

The two centers in the knees, which as we will see are associated with the earthy center at the base of the spine, are assigned to Saturn,

---

[3] Plummer, undated.
[4] Heindel 1938, p. 34.

the earthiest of the planets in astrological symbolism. The genital center is assigned to Mars or Venus, depending on gender, and the planet not thus assigned is then referred to the thymus or, in another and rather more explicit sense, to the sexual partner of the practitioner. The liver and the adrenals are on the same approximate level in the torso, and the liver is traditionally assigned to Jupiter in astrological medicine, so Jupiter goes with the liver center. The throat center, like the thyroid, can only be talkative Mercury, while the two glands and centers in the head can be equated to Neptune and Uranus or, in the more traditional version of astrology that uses only the seven ancient planets, to the Moon and Sun, respectively. As we will see, which of these glands is the Moon and which is the Sun varies significantly from one source to another.

There are interesting parallels to these attributions in George Winslow Plummer's book *Rosicrucian Symbology*, which is teasingly subtitled *A Treatise Wherein the Discerning Ones will find the Elements of Constructive Symbolism and Certain Other Things*. Among the "certain other things" are important indications concerning the inner alchemy of the Rosicrucians. Plummer starts with a point in a circle, divides the circle into four parts with a cross, extends one line of the cross downward, and only very gradually reveals that he is drawing a map of the human body. The dot in the circle identifies the head with the sun, and the symbol of Venus is placed at the genital center— the human body Plummer has in mind is evidently female and is accordingly shown with prominent breasts.[5]

The other planets are not shown, except that Mars appears twice— once at the center of the head pointing downward, and once just above the genital center pointing back up, to represent the flow of sexual energies through the body. A little later in the book, in another, slightly different image of the body with geometrical patterns superimposed on it, a rose is shown blossoming on the vortex at the throat. With the body and outstretched arms forming a cross shape, this establishes the Rose Cross symbol of the Rosicrucian tradition.

CB

In the system of inner alchemy taught by the Rosicrucian Fellowship, the goal of spiritual practice is the redirection of the life force from

---

[5] Plummer 1916, pp. 16–7.

the genital center and sexual expression to the higher centers of the subtle body, and especially to the pineal and pituitary glands. By doing this, the practitioner gains the power to perceive the spiritual worlds *The Rosicrucian Cosmo-Conception* explains this in straightforward terms: "To regain contact with the inner Worlds, all that remains to be done is the reawakening of the pituitary body and the pineal gland. When that is accomplished, man will again possess the faculty of perception in the higher worlds, but on a grander scale than formerly, because it will be in connection with the voluntary nervous system and therefore under the control of the Will."[6]

The publicly available writings of the Rosicrucian Fellowship do not offer any techniques for redirecting sexual energies. A vow of celibacy and ordinary willpower are apparently enough from the Heindel's perspective, at least for beginners. Plummer's approach was at once more nuanced and more forthcoming. In *Rosicrucian Manual*, he rejects the idea that celibacy is necessary for the awakening of the spiritual senses and states that the sexual activities of individuals are their own business, but he also provides an exercise for redirecting sexual energies when their ordinary expression is inappropriate or unwanted:

> At such times as sexual desire seems imperative, stand erect, muscles tense, place the hands palms down over the sex organs—partially or, better still, completely disrobed—and while doing so, concentrate on the thought: "I Will that this power ascend to higher regions—that it follow this path—I can feel it so doing," meanwhile drawing the hands up slowly on each side of the abdomen, following the natural curve of the body, until they stop over the nipples or mammary glands. Pause a moment until conscious of a distinct swelling of the breasts, a sensation of energy therein. Practice this on several occasions until the evidence of the upward surging of the vital powers is undoubted. Then, as a step farther, the next time it is practiced, bring the hands up to the throat, until it manifests in a distinct desire to speak with force and vigor. Third step—bring the hands completely up over the back and front brains, and you will become conscious of a power to create in the line of thought or mental process never before experienced. This practice is invaluable to the men or women who use their brains rather than their hands in the regular occupations of life.[7]

---

[6] Heindel 1909, p. 477.
[7] Plummer 1923, p. 44.

This is not the Sixth Rite that Kelder included in his pamphlet, but it serves the same purpose of redirecting sexual energies, and its ultimate goal is the same: in Kelder's language, to see with the Eye of Revelation. A glance through the occult literature of the early twentieth century will turn up several other practices that differ in approach but have the same purpose. The partial or total reorientation of sexual energies in order to awaken hidden powers in human consciousness was a central theme of occult teachings at that time, and methods for doing this can be found in a great many sources.

Violet Firth Evans, who became one of the twentieth century's most influential occultists under her pen name Dion Fortune, is among the examples here. She included a different exercise for redirecting the sexual energies in her book *The Problem of Purity*, one of her two volumes on the subject of sex and occultism.[8] Her approach involves drawing the sexual energies up through the inside of the spine to the brain. For reasons we will discuss in the next chapter, this was not an approach that American occultists in Fortune's time were willing to risk.

ः

To understand how the process of awakening the inner senses was supposed to work, it will be helpful to start with a closer look at two of the glands in the endocrine system, the pineal gland and the pituitary gland. As already noted, both of these are on the underside of the brain. They were identified as significant factors in human life much earlier than the other glands in the endocrine system, and occultists took note. Both glands, for example, are discussed in detail in Helena P. Blavatsky's private Esoteric Section lessons in 1889, which were issued to advanced members of the Theosophical Society, inevitably leaked out, and became a central resource for occultists for three-quarters of a century thereafter. As we will see, later occultists were not slow to follow up on the hint.

The pineal gland, which is reddish-gray and shaped like a tiny pine cone, is roughly at the center of the head. Place your fingertips right where the top of your ear joins your head on each side, and your pineal gland is halfway between them. About the size of a rice grain, it is richly supplied with blood, more richly than most other tissues in the

---

[8] Fortune 1988, pp. 120–22.

body, and it also has nerves coming into it from all three of the nervous systems in the human body: the central, sympathetic, and parasympathetic systems, which will be discussed in a later chapter.

Though it is located as far from light as anything in the head can be, the pineal gland has the same basic structure as an eye. Evolutionary biologists have discovered that it is descended from a third eye that some of our earliest prehuman ancestors had hundreds of millions of years ago, and some lizards and other reptiles still have today. It has another connection to vision, for the pineal gland is located directly between the two optic thalami, cone-shaped masses of nerve tissue that have a crucial role in processing the nerve signals that arrive through the optic nerves from the eyes.

The pituitary gland, which is dark reddish-brown, is divided into two visible lobes, one behind the other. It is located well forward of the pineal gland, behind the bridge of the nose and between the two temples. By most measures, it is the most important gland in the endocrine system. It controls the hormonal activities of the other glands in the systems, and if it is removed or destroyed, death follows inevitably within a few days. Both the pineal gland and the pituitary gland release their hormones into the bloodstream, and so one can affect the other that way, but they have another, far more direct connection by way of the cerebrospinal fluid.

Few people nowadays seem to be aware that the human brain floats in a pool of its own special fluid. The cerebrospinal fluid surrounds the entire brain and spinal cord and is held in by a tough membrane called the dura mater. It also flows through a series of open spaces in the brain and the spinal cord, which are called ventricles. The main function of the cerebrospinal fluid is to cushion the brain's delicate tissues from sudden shocks, but it also carries hormones and other chemicals from one part of the brain to another. The pineal gland is among the sources of hormones in the cerebrospinal fluid. It connects to the third ventricle, the open space that runs along the midline of the brain, and so it can excrete hormones directly into the cerebrospinal fluid without having to go through the bloodstream. The pituitary gland is also in contact with the cerebrospinal fluid as well as the bloodstream and so can receive pineal gland's secretions by either route.

According to occult teachings, the awakening of the Eye of Revelation depends on this double connection. Under certain special circumstances, the pineal gland excretes a special hormone, the "secret Principle" mentioned in Plummer's lecture on the glands, into the cerebrospinal fluid. This stimulates the pituitary gland as well as the optic thalami and several other parts of the brain. The stimulation of the pituitary gland releases hormones and other chemicals more typical of youth than old age, and these help restore the body's vitality. The stimulation of the optic thalami, in turn, results in the "opening of the third eye" referenced in the spiritual traditions of Asia: the attainment of the ability to see directly into the spiritual worlds.

Discussions of the opening of the third eye in more recent books on alternative spirituality usually equate the third eye with one of the seven chakras, the flowerlike centers of subtle energy, which are located along the spine and brain and described in great detail in Indian esoteric texts. The specific chakra identified with the third eye is the Ajna chakra, which is located in the middle of the brainstem at the level of the eyes but has its reflection in the physical body between the two eyebrows. According to Hiroshi Motoyama's capably researched study *Theories of the Chakras*, the Ajna chakra is in fact associated with the third eye and the pituitary gland.[9] Thus the secret alchemy we are considering appears to have some elements in common with the Indian tradition of the chakras.

Yet the standard Indian methods of rousing the kundalini, the "serpent fire" that rises up the spine to awaken the chakras in kundalini yoga, are not used in the traditions we are exploring. The Sixth Rite in *The Eye of Revelation*, the yogic practice of *uddiyana bandha*, is the one exception, and in classic kundalini yoga, *uddiyana bandha* is a very basic exercise suited to beginners, a preliminary practice leading the way to more important practices such as nauli kriya.[10] Nor do *uddiyana bandha* or any of the other practices central to kundalini yoga seem to have been used by the Rosicrucian orders that taught the secret of the seven vortices or the awakening of the pineal gland. We are dealing with a distinctly different tradition—and thereby hangs another part of our tale.

---

[9] Motoyama 1981, p. 25.
[10] Shivananda 1980, pp. 136–37.

CHAPTER 7

The Chakras

These days, kundalini yoga is a common style of yoga, practiced all over the industrial world. It claims to waken the kundalini, an energy sleeping in a center at the base of the spine, and lead it up through the chakras along the spine to the crown of the head, granting health, happiness, and enlightenment. As with most kinds of yoga in the modern Western world, its clientele is predominantly female and comes from the middle and upper middle classes. Books on the subject, of which there are many dozens, pitch it to potential students as a gentle, nurturing route to physical and spiritual health that anyone can practice without risk. Its techniques are less physically challenging than those of many other varieties of yoga and require only a modest investment of time and effort each day. It's hard to think of anything less threatening or better suited to widespread practice.

With that in mind, it can be a shock to read accounts of kundalini yoga from a century ago. *The Serpent Power* by Arthur Avalon (another pseudonym; his real name was Sir John Woodroffe), the 1918 volume that provided the first detailed English language account of kundalini yoga, presents that system as a demanding and potentially dangerous practice that can only be safely performed under the close supervision of an experienced tantric guru, and even then sometimes results in catastrophic failure. G.S. Arundale's *Kundalini: An Occult Experience*, published in 1938, agrees: "It is clear from all this how complicated the process of the awakening of Kundalini really is, and how foolhardy an individual would be who sought to arouse it without wise sanction, and without a certain amount of guidance. It is almost certain he would come to terrible grief."[1] The same point is made in more recent works: Hiroshi Motoyama's widely respected 1981 manual *Theories of the Chakras* warns: "Please realize that the practices enumerated here traditionally have been taught only to outstanding students under the careful guidance of a guru. Practicing alone from a book can easily lead to a misunderstanding and thus considerable danger. It is essential that the instructions recorded here be followed only under the most expert guidance."[2]

Grasp the details of the practices these books are discussing and it's easy to understand the intensity of the warnings. There is more than one way to work with kundalini—a detail not often grasped by recent Western writers on the subject. All the ones known to me, however, start with the muladhara chakra, which is located at the base of the spine. There is, as already mentioned, an endocrine gland or something like one at that point: the coccygeal glomus, also known as Luschka's gland. It is an irregular oval about an inch across in adults, located below or just in front of the tip of the coccyx or tailbone. Modern Western anatomists don't know what function it serves and therefore tend to call it a vestigial structure.

Indian books on yoga tell a different story. From their perspective, the muladhara chakra contains the most powerful concentration of life force in the human body, the kundalini (from *kundala*, "coiled up" in Sanskrit). In most people, the kundalini remains latent from birth to death, never releasing its considerable power. Certain spiritual disciplines, however, can awaken it. There are at least two things that can be done with it as it awakens. In one of them, the method of laya yoga, the kundalini is withdrawn entirely from the muladhara chakra and drawn up the spine, finally reaching the Sahasrara chakra at the crown of the head; when this is done, the body enters into a deathlike coma but the consciousness, attaining enlightenment, can range at will throughout infinite space. In the other approach, the method of kriya

---

[1] Arundale 1938, p. 30.
[2] Motoyama 1981, p. 109.

yoga, the kundalini remains anchored in the muladhara chakra but circulates up and down the spine, supercharging all the chakras and bringing about enlightenment in a single lifetime. Both these methods thus have ambitious spiritual aims but run serious risks.

The risks are far from abstract. One of the most widely read late twentieth century books on the subject, Gopi Krishna's *Kundalini: The Evolutionary Energy in Man*, describes the author's harrowing experience with a spontaneous kundalini awakening. It left him flat on his back in bed for years, with doctors convinced on more than one occasion that he would not survive the process. Such crises are common enough these days that several networks have been founded by psychotherapists familiar with the symptoms of kundalini activation, with the goal of getting help to people facing the same sort of challenge.

What happened? How did a process so demanding and risky suddenly become safe enough to teach to middle-class suburbanites? As Philip Deslippe explains in an influential essay, the explanation is quite simple: kundalini yoga as practiced in the Western world today has very little in common with the older traditions.[3] The currently popular methods were invented in the middle years of the twentieth century by Harbhajan Singh Puri, who marketed himself to a mostly American audience under the name Yogi Bhajan and became one of the most successful mystical entrepreneurs of his time. Bhajan, as we may as well call him, learned some elements of his system from the Sikh mystic Maharaj Virsa Singh and the Hindu teacher Swami Dhirendra Brahmachari, but he synthesized them into a new and carefully restricted method of practice which differs in almost every way from the older traditions.

The change from the traditional forms of kundalini practice to modern, Yogi Bhajan-derived kundalini yoga is simple enough. In place of the demanding and potentially dangerous methods used in the classic system, today's kundalini yoga uses relatively easy asanas, simple methods of pranayama, mantra recitation, and very brief sessions of the classic *bandhas* (muscular contractions) to produce a gentle rousing of the energy in the spinal centers, in place of the high-intensity effects sought by the older tradition.[4] The purpose of the practice is not the total transcendence of material existence sought by the yogins of an

---

[3] Deslippe 2012.
[4] See, for example, the practices set out in Karena and Khalsa 2017.

earlier generation, but ordinary good health, happiness, and spirituality wholly compatible with life in the world.

Most of these points can be made equally well of the Five Rites, and of the broader system of practice we are exploring. The system of vortices taught by Max Heindel and George Winslow Plummer can best be understood as another response, paralleling Yogi Bhajan's, to the dangers of classic kundalini yoga. Inspired by the example of kundalini yoga but aware of the risks traditionally associated with it, Heindel and Plummer were among a great many occultists who developed and taught safe and effective methods of working with the energy of kundalini from within a Western occult perspective. The seven vortices are far from the only experiment in this direction, and a look over some of the other ventures of the same period will help place the Five Rites in their context.

෪

The most widely used method of this kind was devised in the 1930s by Israel Regardie, one of the most influential figures in twentieth century Western occultism. Born in England and raised in the United States, Regardie began his occult studies as a student of George Winslow Plummer's Rosicrucian order, the SRIA. In 1928, he went to England to study with the notorious occultist Aleister Crowley but left Crowley in 1930 and joined one of the branches of the Hermetic Order of the Golden Dawn.

One of the Golden Dawn's instructional papers, "On the Work to be Undertaken Between Portal and $5° = 6°$," includes an exercise in which the student visualizes the Cabalistic Tree of Life, a diagram of ten circles and twenty-two lines, in his or her aura.[5] Regardie took that exercise and reworked it extensively, drawing on other occult literature of the time, to create what has since become known as the Middle Pillar exercise.

The basic concept of the Middle Pillar exercise is the awakening and empowering of a set of energy centers located in the body. While this sounds like kundalini yoga in the abstract, nearly every detail differs. The current of energy comes from far above the head rather than from the base of the spine, it runs down the midline of the body well in front of the spine rather than up the spinal column, and there are five centers

---

[5] Regardie 2015, pp. 108–16.

rather than seven—one just above the head, one at the level of the throat, one at the heart, one at the genitals, and one at the soles of the feet. The exercise is done standing, preceded by the Lesser Ritual of the Pentagram—the standard preliminary ritual exercise of the Golden Dawn system—and is followed by a process of circulating energy through the aura, the egg-shaped zone of subtle energy surrounding the physical body.

As originally presented by Regardie in his preliminary 1937 essay "The Art of True Healing," and then in more detail in his 1938 book *The Middle Pillar*, the exercise involves no physical movements at all. Breathing, visualization, and the chanting of words of power (the Western occult equivalent of mantras) provide the technical methods that awaken the energy centers in the body. The resulting practice is as safe as Yogi Bhajan's kundalini yoga and, in its own way, as effective. This is why the Middle Pillar exercise, as Regardie devised it or in a dozen or so slightly varied forms, has become one of the standard elements of training in many modern Western occult schools.

Another practice meant to awaken the body's energy centers, less widely known than the Middle Pillar exercises, is found in some occult schools belonging to the Martinist tradition—a movement of Christian occultism founded by the eighteenth century mystic Louis-Claude de St.-Martin—and also, oddly enough, in some schools that use the name and symbolism of the ancient Druids. This exercise, variously called "the Stimulator" or "the Body of Light," involves drawing energy up through the soles of the feet and filling the entire body with it, a little at a time, ending at the crown of the head. It carefully avoids focusing on any of the body's energy centers, so that the whole body receives a gentle recharging with life force. This has also proven to be safe and effective in practice.

Harry J. Gardener included an exercise of this latter type in one of his monographs for beginning students, *The Golden Gate to the Garden of Allah*. His exercise is closely related to the Stimulator, but the light does not well up from the feet; it is generated in the back of the head, in the region of the pineal gland, and cascades down the body into the feet, rising up to fill the body from there. It also involves a systematic tensing and relaxing of the muscles in the body. (It will be described in detail later on, as it is a core element of the exercises we are exploring.)

Certain other practices of the same general type have found a comparable niche in Western occultism. Most of the ones known to me were clearly inventions of the late twentieth and early twenty-first century, inspired by the relatively detailed knowledge of kundalini yoga and other subtle-energy exercises made possible by the publishing boom in occultism and spirituality that followed the 1960s. The Middle Pillar and Stimulator exercises are good reminders, however, that students of Western occultism further back were interested in developing an equivalent of kundalini yoga that could be practiced by individuals without the constant supervision of a trained guru.

The Five Rites, the system of vortices discussed by Heindel and Plummer, and certain exercises included in the writings of Harry J. Gardener belong to another such system. Unlike the Middle Pillar exercise, which was based entirely on the Cabalistic Tree of Life, or the Stimulator, which betrays no knowledge of subtle centers at all, the system of Rites and vortices was crafted by someone who knew more than a little about the chakras and the traditional art of raising the kundalini up the spine. The evidence for this may be found through a careful consideration of the seven vortices themselves.

cs

The system of seven chakras used in most modern Western books on kundalini yoga, and in the much wider range of New Age and occult literature that discusses chakras, is a highly simplified version of a much more complex original. Read texts on kundalini and the chakras by traditionally educated Indian gurus and several points become immediately clear. To begin with, there are many more chakras than the seven usually talked about in Western sources, and the location of some of the usual set is by no means certain: the manipura chakra, for example, is located at the solar plexus by some authorities and at the navel by others.

There are also alternative sets of chakra teachings, just as deeply rooted in Indian tradition, that have different numbers of chakras and awaken them in different ways. (Buddhist schools generally use fewer chakras than Hindu schools, for example, with four as a common number.) India is a huge subcontinent with a very long history, after all, so it should come as no surprise that practitioners in different times, places, and schools should have come up with a rich diversity of theories and practices.

Three of the vortices used in the Five Rites and the Rosicrucian practices linked to it can nonetheless be equated in a straightforward manner with chakras belonging to the standard set of seven. These vortices share not only the same locations as the chakras but the same general functions. The vortex located at the base of the sexual organs, for example, is equivalent to the Swadhisthana chakra, the second in the classical sequence; the vortex located at the throat is equivalent to the Vishuddha chakra, and the vortex located in the front of the head, at or near the pituitary gland, corresponds to the Ajna chakra.

Each of these chakras has specific powers assigned to it, which are said to be mastered by the practitioner who awakens them.[6] The Swadhisthana chakra when awakened grants psychic powers and intuitional knowledge, and overcomes death. The Vishuddha chakra when awakened gives supernatural knowledge of sacred things and also of past, present, and future, and enables the practitioner to survive even the dissolution of the cosmos. The Ajna chakra when awakened brings complete spiritual liberation; Swami Sivananda comments simply enough, "the benefits that are derived by meditation on this chakra cannot be described in words."[7] The focus of the lower two chakras on everlasting life and supernatural knowledge, while colorfully phrased, have much in common with the promises made in *The Eye of Revelation* and the Rosicrucian literature we have explored.

The remaining vortices cannot be identified with chakras in the usual set of seven, but that does not mean they have no connection to the chakra system. While the major chakras along the spine get nearly all the attention in Western books on the subject, Hindu texts record many other, less important chakras. According to some accounts, there are 21 minor chakras and 49 additional chakras in and around the human body. The two vortices in the knees can be identified with one pair of minor chakras, the Sutala chakras.

The Sutala chakras belong to a set of seven paired chakras in the legs, the Patala chakras. These correspond to the underworlds of Hindu tradition, and thus to states of consciousness below the human level. Each of them, however, can be redeemed and transformed into centers of positive energy and sources of superhuman states of consciousness by the process of awakening them and linking them to the higher

---

[6] The accounts here are from Sivananda 1980, pp. 50–7.
[7] Sivananda 1980, p. 57.

chakras. All the Patala chakras are subsidiary to the Muladhara chakra or root center at the base of the spine, but each of them is also paired with one of the higher chakras along the spine. In each case, awakening one of the Patala chakras stimulates the Muladhara chakra and also the associated chakra higher up.

As centers of negative energy and lower consciousness, the knee centers or Sutala chakras are associated with jealousy and a desire for revenge. People who are caught up in the consciousness of the Sutala chakras obsessively desire what others have and brood over what they lack, becoming full of ill will. To overcome the negative consciousness of the underworld of Sutala, it is necessary to cultivate forgiveness and generosity. If this is done, the Sutala chakras become centers of mobility, flexibility, adaptation, and the quality of will that works around all obstacles and cannot be dissuaded from achieving its goals. They also provide an indirect stimulation to the Muladhara chakra at the base of the spine and the Anahata chakra at the heart.

The underworld realm of Sutala has a fascinating place in Hindu tradition. Like the other underworld realms, it is ruled by a demon king, but its king Bali or Mahabali, demon though he is, has an unusual reputation for piety and virtue: he is a noted devotee of the great god Vishnu. His story occurs in many of the classic Hindu texts, including the *Mahabharata*, the *Ramayana*, and several of the *Puranas*. According to these accounts, Bali was so virtuous and devout that he won mastery over the whole cosmos, and Vishnu had to regain it from him by a trick. Because of Bali's devotion to him, however, Vishnu made him immortal, and in the next great cycle of time, he will become the ruler of the heavens. Read this symbolically and it suggests that the energies of the Sutala chakras, if handled with virtue and piety, lead to longevity and a connection with the spiritual worlds: that is, the claim at the center of the tradition we are discussing.

The vortex toward the back of the head is also a known minor chakra, the Bindu chakra. This is associated with the Moon, and it is the source of the *amrita* or nectar of immortality in Hindu tradition. The awakening of this minor chakra is held to bring longevity and good health, and in current Western chakra practice, it is stimulated to banish tension and depression. Here again, the connection with the purposes of the Five Rites is not hard to recognize.

One of the exercises included as a basic spiritual exercise in Harry J. Gardener's writings—the practice related to the Martinist Stimulator exercise mentioned above—draws very explicitly on this detail of Hindu teaching:

> The procedure is as follows: gently massage the back part of the head and neck. This causes the thoughts to proceed to the back of the head. After massaging for a minute or even a little longer, then concentrate quickly (with hands now at side of the body) on the back of the head. Now imagine Universal Energy in the form of a bright, radiant light (let it be any color that comes to you naturally) is being generated in the rear part of the head.
>
> Imagine that Power is forming from within, getting brighter and more radiant. See this force becoming brighter, until the whole back part of the head is filled. Then you release a stream of it, and let it flow down the spine and into the left foot. See with the mind's eye the energy going into the foot. At the same time, tense the foot; continue to let the energy flow and fill the left leg, until the whole leg is filled with the bright light. Every muscle in the leg should be tense.
>
> Next, fill the right foot and leg. Then proceed to fill the abdomen with this light, gradually letting it fill the body, and tensing every muscle as it strikes it. Continue to flood the body with UNIVERSAL ENERGY until it is filled to a level with the armpits. Then start tensing the left arm from the fingers to the wrist, then to the elbow, and then up on the arm to and including the shoulder. Do the same with the right arm and hand. Then continue filling the body from the chest up the left side of the neck and face, then the right side, until the whole body is tense and filled with glorious Universal Energy.
>
> Do this exercise slowly enough so that it requires about sixty seconds' time to accomplish it. After holding it for a minute, start thrilling with health and power. Remember; UNIVERSAL YOUTH completely fills your body. Next, relax the left foot to the hip, then the right foot to the hip, then the body, arms, hands, neck, and face in the same order you. filled them.
>
> Completely relax, but continue to hold the thought of the bright Universal Light and Energy filling your being. Don't turn off the light—let it and the energy remain, but no tension.[8]

The light descending from the back of the head, of course, is the amrita, the subtle substance that brings immortality, which flows from the Bindu chakra when it is awakened.

---

[8] Gardener 1944, pp. 12–3.

All this raises a fascinating set of issues. In 1909, when the system of seven vortices was first published by Max Heindel, not many people in the Western world knew much about the seven major chakras, and minor chakras such as the Sutala chakras and the Bindu chakra were known only to specialists fluent in Sanskrit. In 1933, when Gardener published the first edition of the monograph that contains the exercise just above, that knowledge was still not widely available in the West. Yet the correspondences of the vortices to the chakras, and the presence of exercises among Western occultists working with fine details of those centers, suggest that whoever originally designed the system of seven vortices and set out the tradition behind them had a good working knowledge of Indian tradition and in particular a solid grasp of the intricacies of classic kundalini yoga.

The most likely places for that knowledge to have existed in the Western world just before 1909 were in central Europe. Until the First World War broke out, Vienna and Berlin were two of the world's most important centers for the scholarly study of Asian religions and religious texts. Both cities were also hotbeds of occult study, with thriving communities of occultists associated with lodges of the Theosophical Society as well as many other independent groups. There if anywhere in the Western world, the specialized knowledge existed to assemble an alternative system of chakras that could be practiced safely without the direct supervision of an experienced guru. Neither my reading knowledge of German nor my background in the specialist literature of the time are adequate to chase down this matter any further, but it seems very likely that the seven vortices were among the things Max Heindel brought back with him from his last European trip, and that either Sylvester Gould or George Winslow Plummer received them, probably by way of Masonic connections, sometime not much later.

Both Heindel and Plummer understood that what they were doing was related to the Indian tradition of kundalini yoga and discussed that tradition at various points in their writings. Heindel in particular was highly explicit about the goals of his work: "when the creative fire is drawn upwards through the serpentine spinal cord," he wrote, "it vibrates the pituitary body and the pineal gland, connecting the Ego" (that is, the essential spiritual self of the individual) "with the invisible worlds by opening up a hidden sense."[9]

---

[9] Heindel 1927, pp. 21–2.

In this description, it is possible to see both the similarities and the differences between classic kundalini yoga and the tradition we have been exploring in this book. Heindel is not talking about a method of bringing the kundalini force all the way up to the Sahasrara chakra at the crown of the head and achieving the total transcendence that results once this is done. His goal is the more modest one of opening the Eye of Revelation, allowing the individual to perceive the unseen worlds directly. Seership rather than sainthood is Heindel's goal, and the goal of the broader tradition of practice we are discussing. The higher dimensions of the soul's destiny are pursued in typical Rosicrucian fashion through prayer and the practice of the virtues, rather than through the more exotic spiritual disciplines of the Eastern traditions.

cs

The evidence cited above leaves one vortex unassigned to a chakra: the liver vortex in Kelder's and Heindel's versions of the system, or the spleen vortex in Plummer's version. Some New Age sources on the chakras online nowadays refer to a liver chakra and a spleen chakra, but I have been able to find no trace of these in the classic Indian kundalini yoga literature available to me. They appear to come from a different source.

The Rosicrucian Cosmo-Conception and the writings of George Winslow Plummer both identify the liver and spleen as energy centers, and they share this identification with a great many late nineteenth and early twentieth century occult texts. To understand the role these centers play in occultism, however, it's necessary first to learn something about occult teachings concerning the planes of existence.

In occult writings, the world of ordinary matter and energy we experience is only one of several different planes, worlds, levels, or regions of being. Despite the terminology, these are not separate from one another: all the planes occupy the same space at the same time, in much the same way that light and sound can move through the same space without disturbing each other or the air in that space. Things on each plane are made of the same underlying "stuff," which is called Cosmic Root Substance in Rosicrucian writings; the difference between one plane and another is a matter of density.

The densest of the planes, the physical plane, is the world of ordinary matter as we know it. One step "higher" (that is, subtler and less dense) than the physical plane is the etheric plane or life world, the world of life force; one step beyond that is the astral plane or desire world, the world of dreams, mental imagery, and emotion. There are other planes subtler than the astral plane, but these three are the ones that matter for our present purposes.

Human beings have bodies on those same three planes. Obviously we have physical bodies, the ordinary structures of bones, muscles, organs, and skin we all know so well. Less obviously, we have etheric bodies—that is, bodies made up of life force, which maintain life in the dense matter of our physical bodies—as well as astral bodies, which are made of the even subtler substance of the astral plane and interact with the astral plane in dreaming, imagination, and ordinary thought. Again, these bodies aren't in three different places. The physical body is surrounded by the etheric body, which is shaped like the physical body but an inch or so bigger in every direction; the etheric body is surrounded by the astral body, which is egg-shaped and a foot or two larger in every direction. (The astral body is what psychics call the aura.)

Each of these bodies has a slightly different center. The center of the physical body is the heart—specifically the lowest point of the heart, the location of the seed-atom around which the rest of the physical body is built up. The corresponding center of the etheric body is in the area of the spleen, and the center of the astral body is in the area of the liver. These three form a triangle around the solar plexus, which is one of the two centers of consciousness in the human individual and will be discussed in the next chapter.

All this makes immediate sense of the final vortex in the traditions we've been studying. Heindel's diagram in *The Rosicrucian Cosmo-Conception* is labeled "Currents in the Desire Body"—this latter phrase is his term for the astral body—and so its midmost center is the astral center of the body, located in the liver. Since the focus of Heindel's training program was on teaching students to achieve the ability to perceive the unseen worlds, the focus of his teachings on the astral center of the body makes perfect sense.

The system of practice Plummer taught was more focused on the etheric plane, and so he placed the midmost center in the spleen, the center of the etheric body. In occult teachings, the astral plane is affected by visualization, while the etheric plane is not. Thus it makes perfect sense that Plummer did not encourage students to work with the vortices. Instead, he recommended concentrating on the solar plexus and practicing breathing exercises, the standard method for working with the etheric body. The advanced lessons of Plummer's course also teach students to perceive the inner worlds, but they do this using a different set of exercises with no direct connection to the seven vortices.[10]

By contrast, *The Eye of Revelation*, even though its teachings focus on physical health, uses the liver center rather than the spleen center as its midmost point. Thus it is clearly intended to stimulate the astral body first. That points to one of the missing pieces of the puzzle we are assembling. If the instruction given with the Five Rites focuses on the astral rather than the etheric body, it is safe to assume that at some point—either in the magical lodge to which Harry J. Gardener and his fellow Fraters belonged, or in some other organization that had the teaching before Gardener and Peter Kelder got it—people who practiced the Five Rites also visualized the vortices.

This also makes perfect sense, because the etheric dimension of the work would be handled effectively by the Five Rites themselves, and by certain other exercises widespread in the occult community when *The Eye of Revelation* first saw print. These will be the next topic of our exploration.

---

[10] The exercises Plummer taught were based on the work of the Austrian scientist and occultist Karl von Reichenbach, nd involved observing a strong magnet in a perfectly dark room. Many people who experiment with this find that they can see, and distinguish between, the two magnetic poles in complete darkness. See Reichenbach 1850.

CHAPTER 8

The Inner Sun

While even basic knowledge of the chakras was hard to come by in America in the late nineteenth and early twentieth centuries, the concept of centers of subtle energy within the body was well known to most Western occultists at that time. So were practices meant to strengthen and energize at least one of those centers. The center in question is the solar plexus, and methods of developing its powers played a central role in occult teachings.

The solar plexus is a mass of nerve tissue located in front of the backbone just behind the stomach. The largest single concentration of nervous tissue anywhere in the body outside the head and spine, it is about the size of a cat's brain. Think of it as your "onboard cat" and you understand much of what you need to know about it. Like a cat, it is intelligent and highly perceptive in its own way, but it knows nothing of words, concepts, and abstractions. It thinks in concrete images and emotions, and so it has to be influenced by using mental imagery and emotional states. Like a cat, too, its primary concerns center on basic biological and social drives. Its basic orientation can be politely described as "feed and breed"—yes, there are less polite descriptions—because it encourages the vital organs to carry out their normal functions of digestion and reproduction.

The solar plexus functions as the organizing center of a web of nerve fibers called the sympathetic nervous system, which connects it to all the vital organs in the trunk and gives it supervision over the circulatory, digestive, and reproductive systems. The sympathetic nervous system, unlike most other parts of your nervous system, does not depend on the brain and the spinal cord, though it connects to the spinal cord in numerous places. The sympathetic system runs itself and manages the organs that keep each of us alive. As the largest node of the sympathetic nerves, the center from which many of the functions of the vital organs are managed, the solar plexus deserves the title that was given to it by anatomists more than two centuries ago: "the abdominal brain."

Manly P. Hall's *Man, Grand Symbol of the Mysteries*, a compendium of occult lore about the human body, which we will discuss in more detail later on, accordingly gives the solar plexus a great deal of attention. Hall describes it as the center of spirit in the body and the third sun of the human microcosm, reflecting the influences of the first two suns, the human spirit and the human soul. It is the magic mirror in which the influences of the spiritual world are reflected: a source of wisdom and power if handled skillfully, but it can also become a source of danger to those who accepted passively whatever images were reflected in it.[1] Hall almost certainly learned this bit of anatomical lore from the teachings of Max Heindel during his studies with Heindel's widow, but it can be found in many other occult texts of the same period.[2]

The symbolism of the solar plexus as a mirror of the Unseen had an interesting reflection in the science of psychology. When the concept of subconscious thinking was first proposed in the second half of the nineteenth century, many psychologists made the intriguing suggestion that the solar plexus might be the center of subconscious thought in exactly the same way that the brain is the center of conscious thought. Though the idea has dropped out of fashion in recent decades, there's much to recommend it. The subconscious mind does in fact seem to be more closely linked to the vital organs, the reproductive system, and the basic functions of physical life than the conscious mind—consider the central role of sex, excretion, and other basic biological realities in the subconscious processes anatomized in such detail by Sigmund Freud.

---

[1] Hall 1972, pp. 199–202.
[2] See, for example, Heindel 1927, p. 22.

Occultists in the early twentieth century paid close attention to the latest discoveries about the nervous system and integrated those into their efforts to awaken the hidden powers of the human body and mind. They accordingly took up the concept of the solar plexus as center of the subconscious mind and put it to good use. William Walker Atkinson, the influential occultist whose work we have discussed already, was among those who found research on the solar plexus a source of inspiration. Under his pen name Theron Q. Dumont, he published a book entitled *The Solar Plexus or Abdominal Brain*. It was among the most popular examples of an entire literature of occult anatomy, which surveyed contemporary anatomical and psychological knowledge about the sympathetic nervous system. Atkinson's book provided a series of exercises, some mental and others focused on the breath, that were designed to activate the solar plexus and get it to align with the intentions of the conscious mind.

By the time Atkinson wrote his book, however, a different exercise for awakening the solar plexus had become all but universal in the occult scene. Among the reasons for its popularity is that it is quite simple to perform. Here is version of the exercise given in Julia Seton's *Psychology of the Solar Plexus and Subconscious Mind*, one of the classics of American occult literature:

> Get calm in thought. Our thoughts are the things with which we admit vibrations into our body which produce harmonious or inharmonious emotions. As we think, so we feel, and if these thoughts are harmonious, we respond constructively; if they are inharmonious, then destructive changes begin within our body. Remember that: "As a man thinketh in his heart, so is he."
>
> Get a beautiful constructive thought vibration, then begin the inbreathing of long deep physical breaths, inhaling through the nostrils, and exhaling through the mouth. During each breath keep the thought of love, peace, health, joy, realization and illumination—anything you desire, but choosing always the thought which will awaken within your physical body the finest and highest impulses. With each breath know that you are really drawing from an inexhaustible supply, the energy that will express for you in the things you desire. Feel that coming into your body, through your solar center, is the great ray of infinite creative energy which you in your higher understanding are simply separating into form for your immediate needs.
>
> After a few moments spent in concentration, breathing and meditation, draw a long, deep breath and exhale slowly. Repeat again

and again until you can feel an increasing respiratory sense; then holding the breath without exhaling, forcibly raise and lower the diaphragmatic muscle. Repeat from five to twenty times, releasing the breath as soon as the exercise becomes effort, and inhaling again. Remember, there must be a period in which one does not breathe at all. We simply let the Great Breath breathe through us. First: To think harmoniously and breathe consciously; Second: To breathe deeply holding each breath as long as possible, then releasing and waiting as long as possible before again inhaling; Third: Inhale, holding breath, and massaging solar center with diaphragm, then releasing, and again taking up the ordinary breath.[3]

This practice—drawing in a breath, raising and lowering the diaphragm while holding the breath, and then releasing the breath, all the while holding an appropriate mental state—had an extraordinary popularity in its day. It found its way into the teachings of the Hermetic Order of the Golden Dawn, where it appears as a method of relaxation for initiates who are too tense and "nervy."[4] It also appears in the writings of popular occult authors of the period such as Elizabeth Towne. Like the Five Rites themselves, it represents the simpler and most practical end of an entire body of occult theory and practice, but it has fallen into the same obscurity that surrounded the Five Rites before their revival and still surrounds the seven vortices and the broader tradition of inner alchemy that makes use of them.

ख

In classic American occultism, the solar plexus was not just the physical center of the subconscious mind, though it certainly had that role in addition to several others. It was also believed to be the center through which the life force was distributed throughout the individual's etheric body. In the fully developed theory, which may be found explained in detail in the Rosicrucian texts cited earlier, the life force streams down to the earth from the sun and is absorbed into the etheric body through the solar plexus. (The connection between this theory, the theory of siderism described earlier, and the solar current discussed in de Prati's *Letters on Tellurism*, will doubtless occur to many readers.) From the solar plexus, it streams outward through twelve channels to fill the etheric body with life.

---

[3] Seton 1914, pp. 42–4.
[4] Regardie 2015, p. 110.

All breathing exercises that use deep slow breaths, according to this teaching, help open the solar plexus to the incoming stream of solar vitality. It was with this in mind that George Winslow Plummer taught the initiates of the SRIA to stand by an open window each morning and breathe slowly and deeply, concentrating on bringing vitality in from the cosmos, and also from this perspective that he insisted that concentrating on the solar plexus was more effective than concentrating on the knee vortices. This was partly a reflection of Plummer's focus on the etheric plane, but there is another principle involved. Here as so often in classic American occultism, the safer and more general practice was chosen instead of the more focused and potentially dangerous one, as part of an overall strategy of avoiding potential risks and providing benefits to a diverse range of students who might have little preparatory training.

The same principle seems to have guided Harry J. Gardener's focus on gentle breathing exercises using the solar plexus as the center. Here is one example from his writings:

> *The Exercise:* Place the body in a reclining posture with the head slightly raised on a pillow. Then with your folded arms (forearms) press down over the Solar Plexus, but not so hard that you cause pain, yet with weight enough to make breathing from the diaphragm rather heavy. Release pressure for a moment with each exhalation.
>
> After fifteen minutes of this deep breathing (and pressing the diaphragm—Solar Plexus—down) remove the arms and relieve the pressure, and so recline that you leave the entire body relaxed. Breathe for a minute or two quickly from the *upper part* of the lungs.
>
> Note: When you relax the arms from the pressure on the Solar Plexus they may feel like raising straight up. If they do, hold them straight and up, this will require a very little effort on your part.
>
> This practice causes, first congestion; second relaxation of the Solar Plexus, of the subjunctive (*sic*), or functional part of the Spirit. By intensifying this center (Solar Plexus) this practice will cause creation of Spiritual activity—it is stimulating from the *physical side* that affects the Spiritual by reflex action.
>
> As a physical process *alone* this practice will quicken ganglionic action in the region of the Solar Plexus. By changing your attention to the NEW HEART, which Is located in the immediate vicinity of the Solar Plexus, you will get the sought-after Spiritual results.
>
> To do this, mentally visualize the NEW HEART as having expanded to the Solar Plexus, then change your attention to the Presence of

God in your NEW HEART and gratefully acknowledge THE FACT
that God is present and continuously so, but at first you may not realize
this fact continually. Do not let that bother you in the least, when the
"crossover period" is fully accomplished you will REALIZE that God
(through the Holy Spirit) is always present.[5]

Once again a relatively gentle and low-intensity practice is given in place
of the more intense and more dangerous methods common in Indian
esoteric literature—and the use of deep breathing and focus on the solar
plexus is central to this work.

The practice of exercising the diaphragm with the breath held,
and giving the solar plexus an internal massage in the process, was
considered by many occult authors to be an even more effective way
of relaxing the solar plexus so that it could bring in an abundance of
vitality from the sun. Yet the awakening of the solar plexus promised
much more than access to greater vitality. In the occult writings of
the early twentieth century, in particular, the solar plexus was not
simply a center of energy; it was also a center of consciousness. As the
"abdominal brain," it was capable of certain modes of thought, and
occultists worked at awakening and energizing it in order to increase
their effective brainpower.

The mental activities of the solar plexus are surprisingly well
expressed in popular culture. Most of us know what it means to have
a "gut feeling" about a situation. That feeling comes from the solar
plexus. Untroubled by words and concepts, the catlike mind of the
solar plexus has its own sources of information and its own perceptions,
and it can pass on messages to the more conceptual mind of the brain.
The brain-mind, however, has to learn to silence its constant chatter
and pay attention to the intuitive promptings from below. Many of the
classic exercises of occultism help with this process. Combine these
with internal massage of the solar plexus through some suitable form of
physical exercise, and the occult practitioner gains a valuable source of
intuition and insight.

The mental side of the solar plexus, furthermore, is not limited to
the subconscious mind. It also links into the superconscious mind, the
dimension of human consciousness that rises above consciousness
into the realms of spirit. As Julia Seton pointed out in the book already

---

[5] Gardener 1961, p. 38.

quoted, the solar plexus "is in union with all the unseen metaphysical forces of the universe, and relates our human life with the wisdom of the ages past, and to come."[6] It is worth comparing this theory with the similar views of Carl Jung, for whom the unconscious includes both the subconscious realm of personal repressions and the superconscious realm of the archetypes.

The great difference between Jung's theory and the occult teachings on the solar plexus, of course, is that Jung did not identify the subconscious or superconscious minds with the sympathetic nervous system. That, as already noted, was one of the distinctive teachings of the occult traditions we are exploring. Anchoring the subconscious in the physical structure of the solar plexus gave occult teachers and students a range of possibilities that can't be matched by theories that focus purely on the perspective of thought. Given the equation of solar plexus and subconscious minds, it becomes possible, from within the occult perspective, to work with the hidden dimensions of the mind by way of breathing exercises and physical movements as well as with the mental methods Jung and other psychologists liked to use.

In the fully developed occult theory, which is found in Seton's book and many others, the brain and the solar plexus form the basic polarity of human consciousness. The activity of the brain was often called objective consciousness or the objective mind, since it deals primarily with the world of objects experienced through the five ordinary senses. The activity of the solar plexus was accordingly called subjective consciousness or the subjective mind, since it deals primarily with the subjective experiences of the self.

The great challenge of the occultist is redefined by this theory as the art of opening up connections between the subjective and objective minds, or in a more strictly anatomical sense, between the solar plexus and the brain. The goal of many occult practices was to link the objective and subjective minds and allow the skilled occultist to achieve robust health as well as the capacity to perceive the spiritual worlds directly. Julia Seton, again, expressed the point of the connection between these centers clearly: "Union and conscious relation of these centers of being within us give us health, strength, beauty, and youth on the physical plane, and open the door for Divine revelation to the soul."[7]

---

[6] Seton 1914, p. 9.
[7] Seton 1914, p. 15.

The usual approach to making contact between brain and solar plexus focused on the relatively direct connection between these two at the solar ganglia, a set of nerve centers branching away from the spine a little above the solar plexus. Nerves from the solar ganglia descend directly to the solar plexus. In occult theory, vitality from the sun could be drawn in through the solar plexus, passed from there through the solar ganglia to the spine, and then proceed up the spinal column to the brain. Meanwhile, the force of the conscious will could descend by the same route to the solar plexus. Simple in theory, this was problematic in practice, for the same reason that the awakening of kundalini was problematic: any upward movement of vital energy along the spinal channel risked dangerous releases of energy that could damage the nervous system and ruin the body and the mind.

∽

There is, however, another connecting link between the two great centers, and between the central and sympathetic nervous systems more generally. This is the vagus nerve, also called the pneumo-gastric nerve, which is arguably the most unusual nerve in the body. Most communications between the brain and the rest of the body are handled by the spinal cord, but the vagus nerve is the great exception. The thickest nerve in the body outside the spinal column, it leaves the underside of the brain and goes down through the neck into the trunk, where it spreads out like a tree, giving rise to a wandering, branching thicket of nerves that connect to all the vital organs. One of its branches, furthermore, goes to the solar plexus, and other branches come into contact with most of the other nerve centers of the sympathetic nervous system.

The network of nerves that center on the vagus nerve, in fact, forms a third nervous system in the human body. It's called the parasym-pathetic nervous system, and one of its functions is to override or modulate the functions of the sympathetic nervous system whenever circumstances require that. As mentioned earlier, the solar plexus and the sympathetic nervous system generally have an orientation that can be described as "feed and breed." The parasympathetic nervous system, by contrast, has a basic orientation of "flight or fight"—that is, it directs the energies of the body toward hard muscular efforts in survival situations and draws energy and blood flow away from the vital organs for this purpose.

This is not the only function of the vagus nerve, however. One of its branches descends to the spleen, and specialists in the jawbreakingly named field of psychoneuroimmunology—the science that studies the effects of the mind and nervous system on the immune system—have shown that it plays a significant role in managing immune reactions against illness, and more generally the overall health of the physical body. It is by way of the vagus nerve, for example, that the placebo effect seems to function, allowing thoughts and imagery to heal the body. It is also through the vagus nerve that the nocebo effect, the placebo effect's wicked sister, allows thoughts and imagery to make the body sick.

Many of the occult writers of the early twentieth century, though they lacked the tools of the modern anatomist, were well aware of the crucial importance of the vagus nerve. They saw it as a secret channel that could be used to convey spiritual influences from the brain to the solar plexus and vice versa. Since this knowledge was one of the core secrets of the occult schools that used it, it was inevitably shrouded in symbolism. Thus Manly P. Hall carefully noted that the Greek mysteries included two vessels for divine fire: the thyrsus or staff of the mysteries of Dionysus, which corresponded to the spinal column, and the narthex or hollow reed of Prometheus, with which he brought the divine fire down to earth, and which Hall identified with the vagus nerve.[8]

In exactly the same way, George Winslow Plummer in his book *Rosicrucian Symbology* discussed a certain vertical line descending from the center of the symbolic human figure's head through its body, passing through a "solar center" on the way. He called the line John, in reference to John the Baptist, "the messenger sent before, to prepare the way." He drew a hard distinction between this forerunner in the human body and the creative Word itself, a distinction that clearly mirrors that between the vagus nerve and the spinal column.[9] The line and the symbolism that surrounds it provides the student with a straight-forward image of the vagus nerve descending from the underside of the brain, at the midpoint of the head, into the trunk and its vital organs. As the messenger that "prepares the way," the vagus nerve begins the process of activating the energy centers of the body, a process that is completed eventually by the kundalini moving up the spine through channels already cleared for it in advance.

---

[8] Hall 1972, pp. 202–03.
[9] Plummer 1916, p. 13.

Intriguingly, there is even a text from the early twentieth century that identifies the vagus nerve with the process of kundalini awakening. This is *The Mysterious Kundalini* by Vasant G. Rele, an Indian physician and religious scholar who set out to correlate the teachings of kundalini yoga with the anatomical structures of the human body. His book, published in 1927, presented a detailed argument suggesting that the vagus nerve rather than the spine was the channel by which the kundalini rises through the body to the centers in the head.

He was almost certainly wrong in that claim, as all other Indian sources I have been able to consult insist, by contrast, that the kundalini ascends through a nadi (energy channel) that runs through the middle of the spinal cord. Nonetheless, Rele makes a good case that some of the effects of kundalini awakening can be brought about through the stimulation of the vagus nerve by breathing exercises and movements. His book, though it was published in India, seems to have attracted a great deal of interest in Western countries as well. Manly P. Hall's *Man, Grand Symbol of the Mysteries* is only one of several influential occult books that cites Rele's work.[10]

Writings discussing in detail the role of the vagus nerve in the awakening of the subtle body are hard to find in occult literature. I know of only two writers that do so, and both of them were occultists active in early twentieth century California. One of them, Dr. George Washington Carey, was a quiet, genial physician who wrote some of the strangest works in modern occult literature. The other was Manly Palmer Hall, the grand old man of California occultism in the second half of the twentieth century, who summed up the whole tradition we have been discussing in half-concealed form in one of his many books.

---

[10] Hall 1972, p. 203.

CHAPTER 9

The Third Eye

George W. Carey was born in the little farm town of Dixon, Illinois in 1845, and traveled west with his family on the Oregon Trail in a covered wagon a few years later. Like Harry J. Gardener, with whom our story opened, he spent his youth and early adulthood in the farm country of Oregon and eastern Washington. In 1885, middle-aged and married, he ran the general store in Yakima, Washington, and studied medicine in what was then the usual way, by apprenticeship with a licensed physician. In his time, there were still many competing methods of healing in American medicine, including most of those that now count as alternative health care. One of them, the biochemic medicine of Wilhelm Schüssler, became the mainstay of Carey's budding medical practice and the focus of his later life.

Schüssler's biochemic medicine was an offshoot of homeopathy, which is a complicated subject all its own. The very short form is that homeopathic physicians take substances that cause symptoms of illness, dilute them in precisely measured ways, and administer them in microdoses, to stimulate the body into healing itself: a drug that causes nausea in large doses, for example, will treat nausea when given in homeopathic microdoses. Biochemic medicine does the same thing, but the substances it uses for its microdose medicines are all minerals that are normally found in the human body.

There are twelve of these minerals: calcium fluoride, calcium phosphate, calcium sulphate, iron phosphate, potassium chloride, potassium phosphate, potassium sulphate, magnesium phosphate, sodium chloride, sodium phosphate, sodium sulphate, and silicon dioxide. Diluted to one part per million by homeopathic methods, these cell salts, as they are called, form the medicine cabinet of the old-fashioned biochemic physician.

These and biochemic medicine in general are typically dismissed as sheer quackery by the spokespeople of modern medicine. As noted in an earlier chapter, this is the standard treatment for any healing modality that does not make money for the medical and pharmaceutical industries. At least two things can be said in favor of the cell salts, however. The first is that unlike the treatments used by mainstream medicine in Carey's time, and of course today as well, they cause no harmful side effects. The second is that in practice, they do in fact seem to provide effective symptomatic relief for many common illnesses.[1]

This was the kind of medicine Carey studied. He was apparently very competent at it, too. In 1894, he published a textbook on the subject, *The Biochemic System of Medicine*, which is still in print today. He also founded the Yakima College of Biochemistry, though this closed after a few years due to a lack of students. His whereabouts over the following years are difficult to trace, but the curtain rises again in 1917. By then he was living in Los Angeles and running a health-care firm of his own, the Chemistry of Life Company, which sold cell salts to the public and hosted lectures by Carey on how to use them. That was also the year that Carey published the first of a series of memorably weird books, *The Tree of Life*. The series finally culminated in 1920 with Carey's magnum opus, co-written with his assistant and successor Inez Perry: *God-Man, The Word Made Flesh*.

Whatever else Carey had been doing between 1894 and 1917, it's clear that he had encountered and studied a solid range of American occult traditions and embraced them with the same

---

[1] I have used the cell salts for ordinary home health care for more than thirty years as of this writing, and the results have been generally equal to or better than those from standard over-the-counter medicines.

limitless enthusiasm he earlier directed toward biochemic medicine. He had become a capable astrologer and worked out a table that assigned each of the twelve cell salts to one of the signs of the zodiac. He had studied the Bible, too, and interpreted it in what might be called, with some degree of understatement, a highly original fashion. Carey had also absorbed some of the teachings of yet another California occultist, a man named Hiram E. Butler, who moved west from Massachusetts in 1890 to found a commune north of San Francisco. Finally, Carey clearly knew his way around the secret teachings we have been exploring in this book.

All this came pouring out into the pages of *God-Man*, framed in terms that are remarkably strange even by the standards of occult literature. Carey argued that Christ was not a historical person or a spiritual principle. As the literal meaning of the Greek word *christos*, "anointed," indicates, it is an oily substance that is formed in the body. The name of Christ's birthplace, Bethlehem, literally means "house of bread" in Hebrew, and so to Carey, Bethlehem is the solar plexus, the "breadbasket" of the human body, and Christ is born there once each month, while the moon is in the sign of the zodiac the sun was in at the time of birth.

The vagus nerve also appears in this cascade of anatomical theology. With its many branches, it is the Tree of Life mentioned in the Book of Genesis, and it must be opened to the free flow of nervous influences in order for Christ to descend along it from Heaven, the brain, to be born in "Bethlehem." Once born, if the right things are done, Christ goes to the Jordan River, the channel of cerebrospinal fluid in the center of the spinal cord, to be baptized. His ministry is carried out in an upward journey along that channel from the solar ganglia to the brainstem. There Christ is crucified at the place where the nerve tracts cross from the right side of the body to the left brain and vice versa.

After this crucifixion, Christ ascends through the ventricles of the brain to the pineal gland, and his influence causes the pineal and pituitary glands to rain down "milk and honey"—that is, to secrete hormones—and transforms the optic thalami into the single eye spoken of in the New Testament: "If therefore thine eye be single, thy whole body will be full of light."[2] To Carey, the Christ oil is the material form of the life essence. When it is properly formed and purified,

---

[2] Matthew 6:22.

and affects the glands, the result is robust psychological and physical health, great longevity, and the awakening of the ability to perceive the spiritual worlds.

Unexpected though Carey's terminology is, the ideas that structure his writings are those we have been following in previous chapters. He has simply chosen an idiosyncratic way to talk about them, and a unique way to work with the flow of energies from the solar plexus up the vagus nerve to the pineal gland. He apparently knew nothing of the seven vortices, or for that matter of the chakras, but his biochemical reinterpretation of the story of Christ draws on the same system of subtle anatomy as the one used by other American occultists, with the solar plexus and the pineal gland taking center stage and the vagus nerve and the upper half or so of the spine in familiar roles.

The path he assigns to the Christ oil from the solar plexus to the brain is the same journey halfway along the spine that other occultists assigned to the life force drawn from the sun: from the solar plexus to the middle of the spine by way of the ganglia that bridge the gap between then, and then up the spine to the brain. All this would have been perfectly familiar to occultists in Carey's time.

Ↄ

It is when Carey begins discussing the proper method to produce the Christ oil inside the body that he veers into unexpected territory. His approach, described in detail in *God-Man* and several of his other books, begins with certain firm lifestyle rules. He believed that alcohol was a dreadful poison that would infallibly destroy the Christ oil, and that any form of sexual activity, with or without a partner, wastes the oil by expelling it from the body in the sexual fluids. Strict abstention from alcoholic beverages and equally strict abstention from sex are the foundations of his method. All by themselves, he believed, these steps would improve the physical, emotional, and spiritual health of the practitioner to a dramatic degree. The long history of celibacy around the world does not exactly lend support to this claim, but then Carey was caught up in his own vision of truth and did not always check his facts against the world the rest of us inhabit.

Once these lifestyle changes have been made, at any rate, the rest of the work can proceed. Carey's method draws on his medical training as a biochemic physician and makes use of a particular protocol of cell salt doses. Carey devised a blend of cell salts that contained all twelve minerals in the same proportions they have in the human body; this blend nowadays is sold by homeopathic suppliers under the trade name Bioplasma. One dose of Bioplasma is taken each day to make sure that the body has an adequate baseline of cell salts for health. This is the foundation of the protocol.

To understand the second part of Carey's protocol, it's necessary to know something about one of the basic theories that guided his practice. As noted above, he assigned each of the twelve cell salts to one of the signs of the zodiac. While the sun is in each sign, the corresponding cell salt is activated. If human beings spent twelve months in the womb from conception to birth, every newborn baby would have had all twelve cell salts activated in the prenatal state and would be much healthier than human beings generally are.

Unfortunately, we spend only nine months in the womb before birth, and so each of us is born with an innate deficiency in the natural activity of three or four of the cell salts. Consider, for example, a child born on the first day of spring, just as the sun enters Aries. It was conceived sometime close to the time that the sun entered Cancer nine months previously, and so it has been in the womb while its mother absorbed the solar influences of all the zodiacal signs from Cancer through Pisces. It has not absorbed the influences of Aries, Taurus, and Gemini, however, and so all through its subsequent life, it will need extra doses of the cell salts that correspond to these signs—potassium phosphate, sodium sulphate, and potassium chloride.

Another child born two weeks later will be in a slightly different condition. This child was conceived sometime around the halfway mark of the sun's passage through Cancer, and so it will receive only a half dose of the solar influence of that sign. It will get its full share of influence as the sun goes through the other signs from Leo to Pisces, and it will get a half dose of the Aries influence. So as it grows, the child will need extra doses of sodium sulphate and potassium chloride (the Taurus and Gemini salts), and roughly half as much extra of potassium phosphate, the Aries salt, and calcium fluoride, the Cancer salt.

These extra doses are the basis for the second half of Carey's protocol. Every twenty-eight days or so, the Moon enters the same sign of the zodiac that the Sun was in at the time of your birth. It stays in that sign for a period that varies from two to two and a half days. During that period, if you practice Carey's method, you take three doses of a mix of cell salts determined by your date of birth, so that the Christ oil that forms in the solar plexus during that period will have the solar and mineral influences it would otherwise lack. Maintain the protocol and the other rules of Carey's system for at least three years, and the Christ oil circulating up through your cerebrospinal fluid to the pineal gland sets the transformation in motion.

All this was published in detail in Carey's books, of which *God-Man* was the most explicit, and taken up after his death by his successor Inez Eudora Perry. It promptly became part of the common stock of teachings in circulation in the occult scene in the United States and elsewhere. Plummer's SRIA circulated a chart of the zodiacal correspondences of the cell salts, which is still to be found on the organization's website. Many other occult correspondence courses in the twentieth century passed on some form of Carey's protocol as part of their secret wisdom. It's indicative that all through the century, long after biochemic medicine fell out of common use, old-fashioned health food stores across the United States still carried the twelve cell salts: there were still enough occultists practicing Carey's protocol to make a set of the cell salts worthwhile for the shopkeepers.

Does the protocol work? Anecdotal evidence from people who have followed Carey's instructions recently suggests that the protocol has significant benefits to physical and mental well-being. In his books, however, Carey claimed that his method would result in nothing short of physical immortality. He seems to have borrowed that idea from the occultist Hiram E. Butler, who was mentioned earlier. Butler argued that the redirection of the sexual energies could stop the aging process and result in perpetual youth and health. Carey seems to have come to the same conclusion, though he identified his cell salt protocol as the key to the transformation.

Quite a few occultists in the early twentieth century leapt to similar conclusions and believed that they too had worked out the key to physical immortality. They were, of course, quite wrong, and the proof that they were wrong was the simple fact that they all died. Carey's death came in 1924, at the ripe but not extraordinary age of seventy-nine. By all accounts, he had a robust and healthy old age and was mentally active up until the end. Those are goals worth attaining, but they don't measure up to the standard of his promises. His successor Inez Perry, the co-author of *God-Man* and the author in her own right of several books and a correspondence course on

Carey's system, tried to explain away that failure; she did as good a job as anyone could have, but the fact of the failure remained impossible to ignore.

In a broader sense, that was a large part of what happened to the world of American occultism that gave rise to the Five Rites and the teachings of Harry J. Gardener, George W. Carey, and the other figures we have surveyed in the previous chapters. The lessons they taught in many cases were valuable and worthwhile, but they did not always live up to the extravagant claims made for them. Just as the value of Gardener's teachings was obscured in the eyes of many readers by the repeated failure of his prophecies, practices that had definite benefits ended up neglected because those benefits failed to measure up to the overinflated promises that had been used to market them.

There was another crucial factor in the eclipse of American occultism, however. All those years of borrowing the cachet of Asia for homegrown practices and teachings turned out to have an unexpected potential for blowback once Asian traditions established themselves as a living presence in American culture. Once yoga studios started opening their doors in American cities, pseudo-Asian exercises like the "hatha yoga" taught by William Walker Atkinson were swept aside; once genuine Tibetan teachers arrived in North America, organizations such as George Adamski's Royal Order of Tibet couldn't compete and either redefined themselves in other terms or went out of existence. An entire world of spiritual knowledge and endeavor sank into obscurity as once-thriving orders closed their doors or struggled on with a tiny fraction of their former membership, and thousands of books went out of print.

A very few teachers of Western occultism in America kept going while others faltered and fell silent. One of them was Manly Palmer Hall.

ဢ

Hall was born in Canada in 1901 and came to the United States with his grandmother in 1904. Fascinated with occultism from childhood on, he joined the Theosophical Society in his teens and in 1919 settled in Los Angeles, where he spent the rest of his life. His first years there were punctuated by regular visits to Oceanside, California, where he studied the teachings of the Rosicrucian Fraternity from Max Heindel's widow and successor Augusta Foss Heindel. By 1920, his lively and well-informed lectures on esoteric philosophy had begun to build a following, and his destiny was set.[3]

Hall was a charismatic speaker as well as a profound student of occult literature, and the Los Angeles occult community welcomed him with open arms—and more to the point, open wallets. In 1928, he published his lavishly illustrated magnum opus, *The Secret Teachings of All Ages*, and shortly thereafter founded the Philosophical Research Society (PRS) as a venue for teaching and research into the wisdom traditions of humanity. Donations and speaking fees flowed in, funding an impressive headquarters complex for the PRS and allowing Hall to amass a world-class collection of occult literature. Books and pamphlets, most of them by Hall, flowed in a steady stream from the publishing arm of the PRS, while Hall's weekly lectures became a fixture of the Los Angeles occult scene.

Many other occult teachers and organizations in the United States pursued the same sort of career in their heyday between the two world wars. What set Hall and the PRS apart is that they never stopped. Hall lived until 1990, and he was still lecturing, publishing, and researching until shortly before the end of his life. Hall also cultivated a serious interest in authentic Asian spiritual traditions and was apparently initiated into at least one of them. His book *Meditation Symbols in Eastern & Western Mysticism* includes unusually detailed information about the two great mandalas of Shingon Buddhism, a Japanese esoteric Buddhist sect; very few Westerners had that information in his day. In 1969, he made a pilgrimage to the Koyasan monastery in Japan, the center of the Shingon sect—something else Westerners in his time very rarely did.[4] Shingon Buddhism had a presence in the Japanese-American communities of several US cities in his time, and it was typical of Hall to seek out esoteric wisdom wherever he could find it.

Yet his core interests remained focused on the traditions of Western occultism, including those central to the tradition that we have been following in this book. All through his career, he continued to draw extensively on the teachings he studied with Max Heindel's widow at Oceanside in his youth. His list of the books he recommended for his students to purchase for their personal occult libraries included Heindel's *Rosicrucian Cosmo-Conception* (marked as "of special

---

[3] Sahagun 2008 is a fine biography of Hall.
[4] See Hall 1970 for his account of the pilgrimage.

importance") as well as Plummer's *Rosicrucian Fundamentals* and *Rosicrucian Symbology*.[5] The same reading list, interestingly, includes as its very first entry a good general textbook of human anatomy.

His own work on the occult aspects and possibilities of the human body appeared relatively early in his career, when the currents we are discussing were in full spate. His 1929 pamphlet *The Occult Anatomy of Man* includes brief discussions of the solar plexus, the pineal and pituitary glands, kundalini, and many of the other themes we have explored in this book. His major work on the human body in occultism, *Man, Grand Symbol of the Mysteries*, appeared just a few years later in 1932 and covers nearly all the theory behind the tradition we have been tracing: the solar plexus, the vagus nerve, the pineal gland, the other endocrine glands, and much more of the same kind.

Hall, in fact, seems to have been familiar with nearly all of the traditions we have been discussing. He drew a great deal of his teaching from his apprenticeship with the Rosicrucian Fraternity, as may be expected, but his more than encyclopedic knowledge of occultism drew in many other threads. He cited Vasant G. Rele, the Indian physician noted above who identified the vagus nerve with kundalini, and George W. Carey, whose book *God-Man* Hall studied closely and praised in measured but positive terms. He provided a detailed and accurate account of the seven primary chakras along the spine and the nature of kundalini. He identified the pineal gland as the Eye of the Gods and spoke learnedly, if evasively, about the role of the solar plexus and the vagus nerve in stimulating it to activity.

He did not discuss any of the practices that could put this knowledge to use, however. That was typical of Hall. In his one book of occult training, *Self-Unfoldment Through Disciplines of Realization*, he presented students with basic instructions in meditation and a great deal of solid practical advice on living a spiritually grounded life and left it at that. He believed that the only safe way to teach occultism was to encourage students to learn the theory by studying classic texts of spiritual philosophy and let them figure out the practical side by themselves with the help of whatever spiritual inspirations they were able to achieve.

Whether or not that was the best option is something that students of occultism will have to judge for themselves. Hall himself seems

---

[5] See Hall 1975, pp. 53–3.

to have had no doubts. Throughout a long and productive career, he gave his weekly lectures on occult philosophy and kept writing and publishing books and pamphlets offering inspiration and instruction to his students. In his later life, he had even less to say about occult practice than before, and for good reason. The hints he had dropped in books such as *Man, The Grand Symbol of the Mysteries* seemed to have fallen on ears that were unable to interpret them. By the time he died, the occult teachings he studied and taught had become a closed book even to most occultists.

With Hall, our narrative has come full circle to the place where it began. It was in Los Angeles, long after most of the other leading figures of the golden age of American occultism had died, that Hall continued lecturing and publishing until shortly before his own death in 1990. By then, the other significant figures in our story were long gone: Max Heindel died in 1919, Rudolf Steiner and George W. Carey in 1924, George Winslow Plummer in 1942, and Harry J. Gardener in 1969. An entire world of occult tradition faded out with them or was preserved solely in private libraries and collections of old books. It is only in the last few years, as online archives made a treasure trove of forgotten texts available to researchers, that it again became possible to piece together the broader picture behind the Five Rites and make sense of the hidden alchemy of the nervous system that is embodied in the exercises and the tradition behind them.

CHAPTER 10

The Secret

The quest to uncover a lost occult teaching, as mentioned back in the introduction to this book, requires many of the same skills that a detective uses to solve a puzzling case. Investigators trying to piece together clues to a crime make a habit of writing out lists of what they found and where they found it, to reveal patterns that might otherwise remain hidden in the data. The same habit is useful in this quest as well. We can begin drawing together the different threads of our investigation by listing the sources examined in the foregoing chapters and noting what common elements can be found in each of them. I have left out those things that are only found in one source—for example, the Hay diet in *The Eye of Revelation*—and focused on the teachings that are shared with multiple sources and thus probably belong to the tradition.

The Eye of Revelation by Peter Kelder

- the seven vortices
- a connection between the throat and genital vortices
- the First Rite
- the Second through Fifth Rites

- the importance of clockwise rotation
- washing daily with tepid water
- the redirection of sexual energies
- the attainment of longevity and good health
- the awakening of the Eye of Revelation

The Writings of Harry J. Gardener

- a link with the Rosicrucian tradition
- a focus on the pineal gland or Bindu chakra
- a focus on the solar plexus
- the attainment of longevity and good health

Hindu Secrets of Virility and Rejuvenation
by Emile Raux (Charles B. Roth)

- the Second through Fifth Rites
- a focus on the endocrine glands
- washing daily with tepid water

Development of Mediumship through Terrestrial Magnetism
by Abby A. Judson

- the First Rite
- the importance of clockwise rotation

The Hindu-Yogi System of Practical Water Cure
by Yogi Ramacharaka

- the attainment of longevity and good health
- washing daily with tepid water

The Writings of Max and Augusta Heindel

- a link with the Rosicrucian tradition
- the seven vortices
- a connection between the throat and genital vortices
- five additional points
- a focus on the pineal gland or Bindu chakra

- a focus on the other endocrine glands
- the importance of clockwise rotation
- the redirection of sexual energies
- the awakening of the Eye of Revelation

The Writings of George Winslow Plummer

- a link with the Rosicrucian tradition
- the seven vortices
- a connection between the throat and genital vortices
- five additional points
- a focus on the pineal gland or Bindu chakra
- a focus on the endocrine glands
- a focus on the solar plexus
- the importance of clockwise rotation
- washing daily with tepid water
- the redirection of sexual energies
- the attainment of longevity and good health
- the awakening of the Eye of Revelation

The Writings of George W. Carey

- a focus on the pineal gland or Bindu chakra
- a focus on the endocrine glands
- a focus on the solar plexus
- the redirection of sexual energies
- the attainment of longevity and good health
- the awakening of the Eye of Revelation

Man, the Grand Symbol of the Mysteries by Manly P. Hall

- a link with the Rosicrucian tradition
- a focus on the pineal gland or Bindu chakra
- a focus on the endocrine glands
- a focus on the solar plexus
- the awakening of the Eye of Revelation

No two of our sources have exactly the same collection of teachings, in other words, but the common threads uniting most of them are not hard to spot. Each of the main authors we have examined gathered up a portion of the secret tradition we have been tracing, along with certain other scraps of teaching, and assembled it all into a picture that seemed to make sense. Look at any one of them and the whole pattern is incomplete. Look at them all, and the secret inner alchemy behind the Five Rites comes into focus.

CB

That alchemy has the goal of working with the life force in a safe and controlled fashion, without the need for constant supervision by an experienced guru, and using that force to awaken the hidden potentials of the human brain and achieve direct personal perception of the spiritual worlds. It has three broad stages, each of which can be pursued in several different ways. The tradition we are discussing was always a work in progress, and the schools and teachers that knew about the system seem to have pursued the process of awakening using varying methods—the normal state of affairs in every esoteric tradition.

In the first, preliminary stage, physical movements and concentration are used to stimulate the solar plexus to activity. This affects the whole sympathetic nervous system and results in improved health through better function of all the vital organs. It also strengthens the power of intuition and the ability to use "gut feelings" to help guide action in the world. Continued further, this stage of the practice has an effect on the vagus nerve, allowing a subtle influence to rise through it to the brain. Sustained practice at this level of the work stirs the pineal gland into activity, releasing a hormonal secretion into the cerebrospinal fluid. The pineal secretion is absorbed by the pituitary gland, the master gland of the endocrine system, releasing a further set of hormones that restore some youthful characteristics to the body.

The pineal secretion is also absorbed by the optic thalami, which plays an important role in processing visual stimuli received from the eyes by the optic nerve. The result is the first stirrings of what Peter Kelder called the Eye of Revelation: the awakening of the capacity to perceive the spiritual worlds directly. It would require extensive research into brain function at this phase to be certain, but my hypothesis is that once they are influenced by the pineal secretion, the optic thalami start picking up signals that do not come from the physical eyes, and feeding them on to the centers in the brain that process ordinary vision. One of the benefits of this part of the process is that the student can begin to see the movements of the life force in his or her body. He or she can begin to adjust the practices to avoid problems in the further stages.

This first stage of the work seems originally to have been carried out using movement exercises with the diaphragm muscles, such as the practice included in Julia Seton's book cited earlier. The Rising Call exercise included in Harry J. Gardener's books is a somewhat more intensive development on the same principle. The Five Rites represent a significant further advance on that mode of practice. The Rites work the muscles surrounding the solar plexus more thoroughly than the simpler diaphragm exercises do and have a correspondingly stronger effect on the vagus nerve and the pineal gland. Kelder's injunction to take the Rites slowly and evenly at first is worth keeping in mind here, since the risk of going too fast and overstimulating the endocrine system was well understood in his time.

The second stage brings in concentration on certain centers in the body. Originally, my research suggests, the solar plexus and the pineal gland were the focus of these exercises. The activation of the vagus nerve continues, but at some point in the process, a stronger influence begins to rise from the solar plexus through the solar ganglia into the spinal cord itself, and from there up into the brain. This can be understood as a gentle, low-intensity version of the kundalini experience. The overwhelming power hidden at the base of the spine is not brought into play; instead, less potent forces flow up from the solar plexus, allowing the practitioner to clear away blockages in the upper spinal centers and gain some of the advantages of kundalini awakening with far less risk. Its main focus is not the total transformation brought about by the awakening of the forces of the root chakra, but rather a more powerful effect on the pineal and pituitary glands than the one provided by stimulating the vagus nerve. In this second stage, the Eye of Revelation opens wide.

The seven vortices discussed in the teachings that Max Heindel brought back with him from Europe belong to this stage and represent the same kind of intensification of the basic practices just outlined that the Five Rites achieved over the simple diaphragm exercise or Gardener's Rising Call practice. As we have seen, the seven vortices were chosen carefully to provide indirect stimulation to the Muladhara chakra at the base of the spine and the Anahata chakra at the heart through the two Sutala chakras at the knees, while directly stimulating the Swadhisthana chakra at the genitals, the Vishuddha chakra at the throat, and the Ajna chakra at the third eye, along with the Bindu chakra at the back of the head and the astral body generally.

The third stage involves circulating the life force from the pineal gland through the body as a whole. I have found only one detailed description of this practice, and it comes from Harry J. Gardener: the exercise using visualized light and body tension to bring energy down from the bindu chakra, cited here on page 65. Gardener's version is clearly tied to the older method of working, which focuses solely on the pineal gland. As far as my experiments have shown, however, it is entirely compatible with the more complex method using the Five Rites and the seven vortices.

Continued practice of this third stage may eventually awaken the kundalini in the muladhara chakra and send it on its way up the spinal column to the crown center. Since the upper half of the spine will already have undergone a gradual cleansing and energizing process in the course of the second stage, this would be much less risky than it would be for a beginner, and the guidance of the Eye of Revelation would help keep the process from running off the rails. Nonetheless, there are still inevitable risks involved.

It is by no means certain, however, that every practitioner was expected to go all the way through to the full awakening of kundalini. The basic practices of exercising the diaphragm and concentrating on the solar plexus and pineal gland can be found in a remarkably wide range of occult publications. Some of them were intended for initiates, but others are clearly written by and for people whose involvement in occultism was limited to a little casual practice and a habit of reading inspiring books. The reader of Elizabeth Towne's popular 1907 pamphlet *Just How To Wake the Solar Plexus*, for example, could not expect to learn about the fine details of occult philosophy, or even the vagus nerve and the occult side of anatomy. Towne's sole subject was how to achieve health, happiness, prosperity, and usefulness in the world.

Peter Kelder makes the same point in the pages of *The Eye of Revelation*. It is quite possible to practice the Five Rites by themselves for the purposes of health, vitality, and longevity—many thousands, perhaps millions, of people have done so with good results. Whether you choose to stop there or go on to add the further dimensions of the practice is ultimately up to you.

ೞ

The system of inner alchemy this book has set out is relatively easy to practice, but several cautions are in order. The most important of these is summed up neatly by an old Rosicrucian saying, *festina lente*—"make haste slowly." Rushing ahead with the practices will not get you results more quickly, and it may harm you. Take everything a step at a time, giving your body ample opportunity to get used to each stage of the work, and the results will be better and more reliable in the long run. For the same reason, the whole system of inner alchemy in which the Five Rites have their place is best learned and practiced a step at a time. This is the procedure I have worked out.

Preliminaries

- While the Rites are less strenuous than many exercise programs in common use today, they can put strains on the shoulders, hips, and spine. Preparing your body for the Rites can therefore spare you an injury. If you have physical limitations or are not used to vigorous exercises, a series of simplified exercises leading up to the practice of the Five Rites is strongly recommended. The best of these known to me is given in Carolinda Witt's book and video *The 5 Tibetans* (see Witt 2008 in the bibliography).
- Alternatively, the older and less physically strenuous system of practices to awaken the Eye of Revelation may be practiced in place of the Five Rites. This is discussed in the text above and also given in detail in Appendix 1, pages 135–138.
- Along the same lines, a checkup by a licensed health-care provider is always a good idea before you start any new exercise program, this one included. This is especially important if you are past your youth or in less than perfect health.
- Several readings of Peter Kelder's *The Eye of Revelation*, which is given in full on the following pages, would be wise before beginning the practice. You might also consider reading Manly P. Hall's *Man, The Grand Symbol of the Mysteries* before you begin, to have a clear sense of the theory behind the practices.
- You will need to decide how you want to deal with sexual energies while working with the system. The sources do not agree on what is required here. *The Eye of Revelation* itself, as well as Max Heindel's writings, suggest that celibacy is an important part of the work, providing redirected sexual energy to help awaken the pineal

gland. George Winslow Plummer's writings are more nuanced on the subject, suggesting that celibacy is unnecessary and that you can simply redirect sexual energies when it's not appropriate to direct them to their natural purpose. In either case, the Sixth Rite or Plummer's alternative way of redirecting sexual energies (cited in full on page 53) can be used.

- You will also need to decide what to do about matters of diet. No two of our sources give the same dietary advice. Peter Kelder recommends a simplified version of the Hay diet, in which protein foods and starch foods are never eaten together; Max Heindel insists on strict vegetarianism; George Winslow Plummer forbids pork and veal while allowing other animal foods and recommends a diet high in fruits and vegetables. My experience suggests that any diet you personally find satisfactory will be suitable for this system.

- In addition, you will need to decide whether you want to include George W. Carey's cell salt protocol as part of your work. Full details of the protocol are given in Appendix 2 on pages 139–144; if you intend to use it, you will need to buy the necessary cell salts in advance.

- Finally, there is the question of potential compatibility issues between the systems discussed in this book and other forms of occult training and spiritual practice, if you practice these. The Five Rites themselves seem to be compatible with almost anything. I have talked to dozens of people who practice them and who also practice a very wide range of other occult and spiritual systems.

- The more advanced levels of the system, however, may not be so compatible with other practices. While experimentation is necessary here, I would encourage practitioners to be careful about going beyond the first stage of the work given below while practicing kundalini yoga, the Middle Pillar exercise, the Taoist lesser or greater circulations of qi, or any other practice that works with specific energy centers and flows within the body. On the other hand, the Martinist and Druid exercise mentioned earlier, the Stimulator or Body of Light, does not focus on any specific centers and seems to be entirely compatible with the work with the seven vortices.

- Once you have assessed these points and made the arrangements you choose, you can move onto the first stage of the practice.

Stage One

- Begin practicing three repetitions of the Five Rites daily. After a minimum of one week, when three repetitions of all five of the Rites seem easy, add two more repetitions of each Rite. Proceed in the same way, adding two repetitions after a minimum of a week, once the current set seems easy. Proceed to the maximum of twenty-one repetitions. If it takes you a year or more to get there, that's fine.

- If one of the Rites gives you more trouble than the others, and you need to add repetitions at a slower pace on that Rite, don't push the other Rites at a faster pace: if you can only do seven repetitions of one Rite, say, limit yourself to seven repetitions of each of them. As the tortoise proved to the hare in the famous story, slow and steady wins the race.

- Wash your entire body once each day with cool or tepid water—not hot, and not cold. The method of washing is up to you: tub bath, shower, or sponge or washcloth bath are all mentioned as options in the sources and seem to be equally effective.

- Spend five minutes each day concentrating on your solar plexus. To do this, sit in any position that leaves your spine relatively straight and supported only by your own muscles. Lotus posture or any other standard Indian meditation posture is suitable. So is the seiza posture used in Japanese martial arts and esoteric practices, which is done by kneeling with the feet stretched out flat, and then sitting back on your heels. So is the standard Western meditation posture, sitting in a chair with your feet flat on the floor, the seat far enough forward that your back does not touch the back of the chair, and the hands palm down on the thighs a little back from the knees.

- Once you settle into the position, relax all the muscles that you don't need to maintain the position, then turn your attention to your solar plexus and breathe slowly, steadily, and gently while imagining a sphere of pale golden light a few inches across in the solar plexus. See and feel it radiating light all through your body.

- When you have reached twenty-one repetitions of each Rite once per day, you are ready to go on to the next stage if you choose to. Alternatively, you may remain at the first stage as long as you prefer. Twenty-one repetitions of the Five Rites and regular practice of the body wash and solar plexus concentration will do very well all by themselves as an exercise program for physical, mental, and spiritual well-being.

Stage Two

- Maintain your daily practice of twenty-one repetitions of the Five Rites. Consider adding a second session each day—for example, if you practice the Rites every morning, you might do your second session in the evening. If you do this, begin with three repetitions of each Rite in the second session and add more repetitions at a maximum rate of two each week. Take as much time as you need. If you choose to add the second session, your goal should be to do a total of forty-two repetitions of the Rites every day, twenty-one in one session and twenty-one in the other. This should be your maximum work with the Rites. If you feel a need for more exercise than this will provide, consider joining a gym or taking up some other form of exercise to do alongside the Five Rites.
- Continue washing your entire body in cool or tepid water once each day.
- In place of the concentration on the solar plexus, begin the process of visualizing the seven vortices. Start by taking the same sitting position you used for the solar plexus concentration. Instead of focusing on the solar plexus, however, turn your attention to your knees. Imagine that behind the kneecap of each knee, inside the joint, there is a little sphere of brilliant white light like a star. Imagine both these points beginning to rotate clockwise. **Please note:** "clockwise" here has the same sense it does in the First Rite; if there was a big clock face laid out on the floor beneath you, the points of light would turn in the same direction as the clock hands.
- Once each day, concentrate on the vortices inside the knee joints—vortices F and G, as Peter Kelder calls them in his booklet—for the time that it takes you to breath seven slow, gentle, even breaths. While concentrating, continue to imagine them as starlike points of light, spinning clockwise. Keep working on the knee vortices, without proceeding to any of the others, until you feel a definite movement of energy in the vortices. How this is experienced varies from person to person; you may sense it as warmth, coolness, a sensation of movement, or in some other way. The important thing is that you feel *something* present in the knee vortices that was not there before.

As you continue your daily practices, you will feel it more reliably and intensely.

- When, and only when, you reliably feel the life force flowing in the knee centers, add the genital center to your daily practice, in this way: concentrate on the knee centers for three, rather than seven, slow, gentle, even breaths. Then, leaving the knee centers, concentrate on the genital center for seven breaths of the same kind. Imagine it as a starlike sphere of light, rotating clockwise, located just above and inward from the base of the penis or clitoris. If you can avoid sexual thoughts or fantasies while doing this phase of the concentration, the awakening of the center will take place sooner.

- In the same way, once you reliably feel the life force flowing in both the knee centers and the genital center, go on to awaken the liver center. Concentrate for three breaths on the knee centers, and then for three breaths on the genital center, and then proceed to concentrate for seven breaths on the liver center, which is located inside the right side of the torso just below the ribcage. Visualize it the same way as the others.

- Proceed in turn to do the same thing with the throat center, the pineal center, and the pituitary center in turn. The throat center is just inside the notch at the middle of the collarbone; the pineal center is directly between the upper part of the ears, toward the back of the head, and the pituitary center is directly between the temples, toward the front of the head. In each case, the center you are awakening receives seven breaths, and the ones you have awakened receive three breaths each.

- Once you have gotten a distinct sense of the life force moving in all seven centers, continue to concentrate on them every day, giving three breaths to each of them (counting the knee centers as a single center) and imagining them as little spinning spheres of light. This, along with the Five Rites and the wash with tepid or cool water, becomes your daily practice. The concentration on the vortices may be performed with good results before or after any meditation practice you may have.

Stage Three

- Once you have made a regular daily routine of all the above, add the following steps, which are done in sequence right after you have finished your daily period of concentrating on the seven vortices.

- Using both hands, gently massage the back of the head and neck for a minute or so.
- Concentrate again on the pineal gland center. Imagine it as a radiant star filling the back of your head with its light. The light may be of any color that occurs to you naturally.
- Imagine the light flowing down your spinal column all the way to the base of your spine, then over to your left leg and all the way down to the sole of your left foot. Imagine the light pooling there, as though it is filling your leg up from the bottom of your sole. As the light fills your foot, tense every muscle in your foot; as it fills your lower leg, tense every muscle there; as it fills your thigh, tense every muscle there, until your entire left leg from hip to toes is tensed and full of light.
- Do exactly the same thing with the right leg, sending a current of light from your pineal gland down your spine to the base and then over and down to the sole of your right foot, tensing your right leg a little at a time as it fills with light. Keep your left leg tense as you do this.
- Do the same thing to your torso from the base up to the level of the armpits, filling it with light and tensing the muscles. Then send the current of light down your left arm to the fingertips, filling the arm a little at a time with light and tensing the muscles. Then do the same thing with your right arm. Finally, bring the light up to fill your shoulders, your neck, and your head and face, tensing these as well. By the time the light reaches the crown of your head, your entire body should be tense from top to bottom.
- Relax the tensions in the order you established them, beginning with the left foot and leg, then the right foot and leg, then the torso to the armpits, and so on. As you relax them, keep the awareness of the light filling your body. As you end this phase, your muscles are relaxed and your whole body is full of the light that radiated from your pineal gland. This completes the practice; take a few slow even breaths and then go about the rest of your day.

It is crucial, as you proceed with the work, not to try to force the movement of the life force from the solar plexus up through the solar ganglia to the spine. This should be allowed to happen spontaneously, and it will happen once the body is ready for it. Force it to happen and you risk a less intense but still dangerous equivalent of the trouble with kundalini that put Gopi Krishna flat on his back for years. When your system is ready, the flow from the solar plexus up the spine will begin by itself.

In exactly the same way, do not do anything with the center at the base of the spine. Let the gentle descending energy that flows through your spine from your pineal gland gradually clear out your spinal channel and stir the root chakra into activity. Through this practice, the way will be made clear for kundalini to flow effortlessly upward in due time. Meanwhile, you will receive all the benefits of the activation of the seven vortices and the hormonal products of the pineal and pituitary glands, and of the gradual opening and cleansing of the spinal channel—to say nothing of the more robust physical benefits of daily practice of the Five Rites.

Many people want to know how long the work will take to yield results. It is only fair to note that this is not a practice that yields instant gratification. How long you will have to keep working to open the Eye of Revelation is a complex matter that appears to depend on personal factors, but months or years will likely be required. Improvements in health and vigor, however, are likely to show up within weeks of beginning the Five Rites, and the exercises of the basic stage will also begin the process of putting you into contact with your solar plexus and teaching you to attend to the nonverbal perceptions of your "onboard cat." Take it a step at a time, repeating the daily practices patiently without interruption, and if the experiences of others are anything to go by, the secret of the Five Rites will become the secret of your own vitality, longevity, and spiritual awakening.

The Eye of Revelation
by Peter Kelder (1939)

Foreword

The Eye of Revelation is truly a revelation. It reveals to you information which has been known and used by men in far-distant lands for centuries. It is information which has been thoroughly tried and tested. Information that will stem the tide of premature old age with its attendant weaknesses and senility. This is information for which Ponce de Leon, and thousands of others down through the ages, would have given all they possessed.

The Eye of Revelation will often produce remarkable mental and physical changes within a month. So much so, in fact, that one gains new hope and enthusiasm, with which to carry on. However, the greatest results come after the tenth week. When you stop to consider that the average person has endured his afflictions from 20 to 30 years to obtain gratifying results in such a short time as weeks sounds almost miraculous.

As long as you live and practice *The Eye of Revelation*, you will get more and still more gratifying results.

Most important: The information given in *The Eye of Revelation* was, for centuries, confined strictly to men. Now, to the surprise and delight of all concerned, it has been found that women, too, get equally beneficial and amazing results. Now man or woman can go on to grand and glorious things, regardless of environment or circumstances.

Get started at once on the marvelous work of youthification, and may success, health, energy, power, vigor, virility, and Life dog your footsteps forever.

THE MID-DAY PRESS

1939

Part One

One afternoon I dropped into the Travelers Club to escape a sudden shower, and while seated in an easy chair waiting for it to clear up, I fell into a conversation with a most interesting old gentleman; one who, although I did not know it then, was destined to change the whole course of my life. I call him an old man for that is exactly what he was. In his late sixties, he looked every year his age. He was thin and stooped, and when he walked leaned heavily on his cane.

It developed that he was a retired British army officer, who had likewise seen service in the diplomatic corps of the Crown. There were few accessible places on the globe to which Colonel Bradford, as I shall call him, although that was not his true name, had not, at some time or other in his life, paid a visit, and warming under my attention he related incidents in his travels which were highly entertaining. Needless to say, I spent an interesting and profitable afternoon listening to him. This was some years ago. We met often after that and got along famously. Many evenings, either at his quarters or at mine, we discussed and discoursed until long past midnight.

It was on one of these occasions I became possessed of a feeling that Colonel Bradford wanted to tell me something of importance. Something close to his heart which was difficult for him to talk about. By using all the tact and diplomacy at my command, I succeeded in making him understand that I should be happy to help him in any way possible, and that if he cared to tell me what was on his mind, I would keep it in strict confidence. Slowly at first, and then with increased trust he began to talk.

While stationed in India some years ago, Colonel Bradford, from time to time, came in contact with wandering natives from the remote fastnesses of the country. He heard many interesting tales of the life and customs of the country. One story, which interested him strangely, he heard quite a number of times, and always from natives who inhabited a particular district. Those from the other districts seemed never to have heard it.

It concerned a group of Lamas or Tibetan priests who, apparently, had discovered "The Fountain of Youth." The natives told of old men who had mysteriously regained health and strength, vigor and virility shortly after entering a certain lamasery; but where this particular place was none seemed exactly to know.

Like so many other men, Colonel Bradford had become old at 40 and had not been getting any younger as the years rolled by. Now the more he heard this tale of "The Fountain of Youth," the more he became convinced that such a place and such men actually existed. He began to gather information on directions, character of the country, climate, and various other tidbits that might help him locate the spot; for from then on there dwelt in the back of his mind a desire to find this "Fountain of Youth."

This desire, he told me, had now grown so powerful that he had determined to return to India and start in earnest a quest for the retreat of these young-old men, and he wanted me to go with him. Frankly, by the time he had finished telling me this fantastic story, I, too, was convinced of its truth and was half-tempted to join him, but finally decided against it.

Soon he departed, and I consoled myself for not going with the thought that perhaps one should be satisfied to grow old gracefully; that perhaps the Colonel was wrong in trying to get more out of life than was vouchsafed to other men. And yet-a Fountain of Youth!!! What a thrilling idea it was! For his own sake I hoped that the old Colonel might find it.

Months passed. In the press of every-day affairs, Colonel Bradford and his "Shangri-La" had grown dim in my memory, when one evening on returning to my apartment, there was a letter in the Colonel's own handwriting. He was still alive! The letter seemed to have been written in joyous desperation. In it he said that in spite of maddening delays and setbacks he actually was on the verge of finding the "Fountain." He gave no address.

It was more months before I heard from him again. This time he had good news. He had found the "Fountain of Youth!" Not only that but he was bringing it back to the States with him and would arrive within the next two months. Practically, four years had elapsed since I had last seen the old man. Would he have changed any, I wondered? He was older, of course, but perhaps no balder, although his stoop might have increased a little. Then the startling idea came to me that perhaps this "Fountain of Youth" might really have helped him. But in my mind's eye, I could not picture him differently than I had seen him last, except perhaps a little older.

One evening I decided to stay at home by myself and catch up on my reading, maybe write a few letters. I had just settled down to comfortable reading when the telephone rang.

"A Colonel Bradford to see you, sir," said the desk clerk.

"Send him up," I shouted, and casting the book aside, I hastened to the door. For a moment I stared, and then with dismay I saw that this was not Colonel Bradford but a much younger person.

Noting my surprise the man said, "Weren't you expecting me?"

"No," I confessed. "I thought it would he an old friend of mine, a Colonel Bradford."

"I came to see you about Colonel Bradford, the man you were expecting," he answered.

"Come in," I invited.

"Allow me to introduce myself," said the stranger, entering. "My name is Bradford."

"Oh, you are Colonel Bradford's son," I exclaimed. "I have often heard him speak of you. You resemble him somewhat."

"No, I am not my son," he returned. "I am none other than your old friend, Colonel Bradford, the old man who went away to the Himalayas."

I stood in incredulous amazement at his statement. Then it slowly dawned upon me that this really was the Colonel Bradford whom I had known; but what a change had taken place in his appearance. Instead of the stooped, limping, sallow old gentleman with a cane, he was a tall, straight, ruddy complexioned man in the prime of life. Even his hair, which had grown back, held no trace of grey.

My enthusiasm and curiosity knew no bounds. Soon I was plying him with questions in rapid-fire order until he threw up his hands.

"Wait, wait," he protested, laughingly. "I shall start at the beginning and tell you all that has happened." And this he proceeded to do.

Upon arriving in India, the Colonel started directly for the district in which lived the natives who had told of "The Fountain of Youth." Fortunately, he knew quite a bit of their language. He spent several months there, making friends with the people and picking up all the information he could about the Lamasery he sought. It was a long, slow process, but his shrewdness and persistence finally brought him to the coveted place he had heard about so often but only half believed existed.

Colonel Bradford's account of what transpired after being admitted to the Lamasery sounded like a fairy tale. I only wish that time and space permitted me to set down here all of his experiences; the interesting practices of the Lamas, their culture, and their utter indifference to the work-a-day world. There were no real old men there. To his surprise, the Lamas considered Colonel Bradford a quite novel sight, for it had been a long time since they had seen anyone who looked as old as he. The Lamas good-naturedly referred to the Colonel as "The Ancient One."

"For the first two weeks after I arrived," said the Colonel, "I was like a fish out of water. I marvelled at everything I saw, and at times could hardly believe what my eyes beheld. I soon felt much better, was sleeping like a top every night, and only used my cane when hiking in the mountains.

"A month after I arrived I received the biggest surprise of my life. In fact, I was quite startled. It was the day I entered for the first time, a large, well-ordered room which was used as a kind of library for ancient manuscripts. At one end of the room was a full-length mirror. It had been over two years since I had last seen my reflection so with great curiosity I stepped in front of the glass.

"I stared in amazement, so changed was my appearance. It seemed that I had dropped 15 years from my age. It was my first intimation that I was growing younger; but from then on I changed so rapidly that it was apparent to all who knew me. Soon the honorary title of 'The Ancient One' was heard no more."

A knock at the door interrupted the Colonel. I opened it to admit a couple of friends from out of town who had picked this most inauspicious time to spend a sociable evening with me. I hid my disappointment and chagrin as best I could and introduced them to Colonel Bradford. We all chatted together for a while and then the Colonel said, rising, "I am sorry that I must leave so early, but I have an appointment with an old friend who is leaving the city tonight. I hope I shall see you all again shortly."

At the door he turned to me and said, softly, "Could you have lunch with me tomorrow? I promise, if you can do so you shall hear all about 'The Fountain of Youth.'"

We agreed as to the time and place to meet and the Colonel departed. As I returned to the living room, one of my friends remarked,

"That is certainly a most interesting man, but he looks awfully young to be retired from army service."

"How old do you suppose he is?" I asked.

"Well, he doesn't look forty," answered my friend, "but from the experiences he has had I suppose he must be that old."

"Yes, he's all of that," I said evasively, and deftly turned the conversation into another channel. I thought it best to arouse no wonderment regarding the Colonel until I knew what his plans were.

The next day, after having lunch together, we repaired to the Colonel's room in a nearby hotel, and there at last he told me about "The Fountain of Youth."

"The first important thing I was taught after entering the Lamasery," he began, "was this." The body has seven centers which, in English, could be called Vortexes. These are kind of magnetic centers. They revolve at great speed in the healthy body, but when slowed down—well, that is just another name for old age, ill-health, and senility.

"There are two of these Vortexes in the brain; one at the base of the throat; another in the right side of the body above the waistline; one in the sexual center; and one in each knee.

"These spinning centres of activity extend beyond the flesh in the healthy individual, but in the old, weak, senile person they hardly reach the surface, except in the knees. The quickest way to regain health, youth, and vitality is to start these magnetic centres spinning again.

"There are but five practices that will do this. Any one of them will be helpful, but all five are usually required to get glowing results. These five exercises are really not exercises at all, in the physical culture sense. The Lamas think of them as 'Rites,' and so instead of calling them exercises or practices, we too, shall call them Rites."

There are SEVEN Psychic Vortexes in the physical body. They are located as follows:

Vortex "A" is located within the forehead.
Vortex "B" is located in the posterior part of the brain.
Vortex "C" is in the region of the throat at the base of the neck.
Vortex "D" is located in the right side of the body above the waistline.
Vortex "E" is located in the reproductive anatomy, and it is directly connected with Vortex "C" in the throat.
Vortexes "F" and "G" are located one in either knee.

These Psychic Vortexes revolve at great speed. When all are revolving at high speed and at the same rate of speed, the body is in perfect health. When one or more of them slow down, old age, loss of power, and senility set in.

Rite Number One

"The first Rite," continued the Colonel "is a simple one. It is for the express purpose of speeding up the Vortexes. When we were children we used it in our play. It is this: Stand erect with arms outstretched, horizontal with the shoulders. Now spin around until you become slightly dizzy. There is only one caution: you must turn from left to right. In other words, if you were to place a clock or

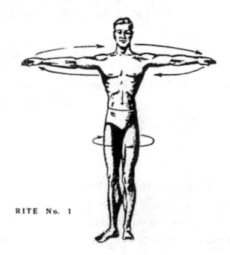

RITE No. 1

watch on the floor face up, you would turn in the same way the hands are moving.

"At first the average adult will only be able to 'spin around' about a half-dozen times until he becomes dizzy enough to want to sit or lie down. That is just what he should do, too. That's what I did. To begin with, practice this Rite only to the point of slight dizziness. As time passes and your Vortexes become more rapid in movement through this and other Rites, you will be able to practice it to a greater extent.

"When I was in India it amazed me to see the Maulawiyah, or as they are more commonly known, the Whirling Dervishes, almost unceasingly spin around and around in a religious frenzy. Rite Number One recalled to my attention two things in connection with this practice. The first was that these Whirling Dervishes always spun in one direction-from left to right, or clockwise. The second was the virility of the old men; they were strong, hearty, and robust. Far more so than most Englishmen of their age.

"When I spoke to one of the Lamas about this, he informed me that while this whirling movement of the Dervishes did have a very beneficial effect, yet it also had a devastating one. It seems that a long siege of whirling stimulates into great activity Vortexes 'A,' 'B,' and 'E.' These three have a stimulating effect on the other two—'C' and 'D.' But due to excessive leg action the Vortexes in the knees—'E' and 'G'— are over-stimulated and finally so exhausted that the building up of the Vital Forces along with this tearing down causes the participants to experience a kind of 'psychic jag' which they mistake for something spiritual, or at least religious.

"However," continued the Colonel, "we do not carry the whirling exercise to excess. While the whirling Dervishes may spin around hundreds of times, we find that greater benefit is obtained by restricting it to about a dozen or so times, enough so that Rite Number One can stimulate all the Vortexes to action."

Rite Number Two

"Like Rite Number One," continued the Colonel, "this second one is for further stimulating to action the Seven Vortexes. It is even simpler than the first one. In Rite Number Two one first lies flat on his back on the floor or on the bed. If practiced on the floor, one should use a rug or

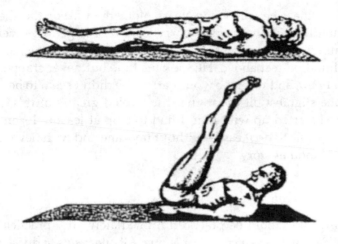

RITE No. 2

blanket under him, folded several times in order that the body will not come into contact with the cold floor. The Lamas have what might be called in English a 'prayer rug.' It is about two feet wide and fully six feet long. It is fairly thick and is made from wool and a kind of vegetable fibre. It is solely for the purpose of insulation, and so has no other value. Nevertheless, to the Lamas everything is of a religious nature, hence their name for these mats—'prayer rugs.'

"As I said, one should lie full length on his 'prayer rug' or bed. Then place the hands flat down alongside the hips. Fingers should be kept close together with the fingertips of each hand turned slightly toward one another. The feet are then raised until the legs are straight up. If possible, let the feet extend back a bit over the body, toward the head; but do not let the knees bend. Then, slowly lower the feet to the floor and for a moment allow all muscles to relax. Then perform this Rite all over again.

"One of the Lamas told me that when he first attempted to practice this simple Rite he was so old, weak, and decrepit that he couldn't possibly lift up both legs. Therefore he started out by lifting the thighs until the knees were straight up, letting the feet hang down. Little by little, however, he was able to straighten out his legs until at the end of three months he could raise straight with perfect ease.

"I marveled at this particular Lama," said the Colonel, "when he told me this. He was then a perfect picture of health and youth, although I knew he was many years older than I. For the sheer joy of exerting himself, he used to carry a pack of vegetables weighing fully a hundred pounds on his back, from the garden to the Lamasery, several hundred feet above. He took his time but never stopped once on the way up, and when he would arrive he didn't seem to be experiencing the slightest bit of fatigue. I marveled greatly at this, for the first time I started up with him, I had to stop at least a dozen times. Later I was able to do it easily without my cane and with never a stop, but that is another story."

Rite Number Three

"The third Rite should be practiced immediately after practicing Rite Number Two. It, too, is a very simple one. All one needs to do is to kneel on his 'prayer rug,' place his hands on his thighs, and lean forward as far as possible with the head inclined so that the chin rests on the chest. Now lean backward as far as possible; at the same time the head should be lifted and thrown back as far as it will go. Then bring the

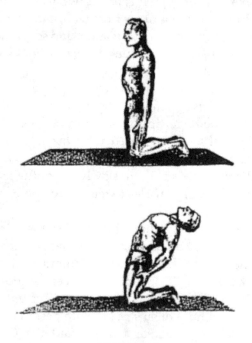

RITE No. 3

head up along with the body. Lean forward again and start the rite all over. This Rite is very effective in speeding up Vortexes 'E,' 'D,' and 'C'; especially 'E.'

"I have seen more than 200 Lamas perform this Rite together. In order to turn their attention within, they closed their eyes. In this way they would not become confused by what others were doing and thus have their attention diverted.

"The Lamas, more than two and a half millenniums ago, discovered that all good things come from within. They discovered that every worthwhile thing must have its origin within the individual. This is something that the Occidental has never been able to understand and comprehend. He thinks, as I did, that all worthwhile things must come from the outside world.

"The Lamas, especially those at this particular Lamasery, are performing a great work for the world. It is performed, however, on the astral plane. This plane, from which they assist mankind in all quarters of the globe, is high enough above the vibrations of the world to be a powerful focal point where much can be accomplished with little loss of effort.

"Some day the world will awaken in amazement to what the unseen forces—the Forces of Good—have been doing for the masses. We who take ourselves in hand and make new creatures of ourselves in every imaginable way, each is doing a marvelous work for mankind everywhere. Already the efforts of these advanced individuals are being welded together into One Irresistible Power. A new day is dawning for the world—it is already here. But it is only through individuals like the Lamas, and you and me that the world can possibly be helped.

"Most of mankind, and that includes those in the most enlightened countries, like America and England, is still in the darkest of the Dark Ages. However, they are being prepared for better and more glorious things, and as fast as they can be initiated into the higher life, just that fast will the world be made a better place in which to live."

Rite Number Four

"Now for Rite Number Four," said the Colonel. "The first time I tried this it seemed very difficult, but after a week it was as simple to do as any of the others.

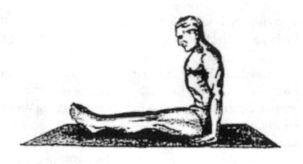

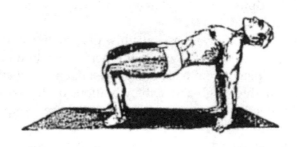

RITE No. 4

"Sit on the 'prayer rug' with the feet stretched out in front. Then place the hands alongside the body. Now raise the body and bend the knees so that the legs, from the knees down, are practically straight up and down. The arms, too, will be straight up and down while the body, from the shoulders to the knees, will be horizontal. Before pushing the body to a horizontal position, the chin should be well down on the chest. Then, as the body is raised, the head should be allowed to drop gently backward as far as it will go. Next, return to a sitting position and relax for a moment before repeating the procedure. When the body is pressed up to the complete horizontal position, tense every muscle in the body. This will have a tendency to stimulate Vortexes 'F,' 'G,' 'E,' 'D' and C.'

"After leaving the Lamasery," continued Colonel Bradford, "I went to a number of the larger cities in India, and as an experiment conducted classes for both English people and natives. I found that the older members of either felt that unless they could perform a Rite perfectly, right from the beginning, they believed no good could come from it.

I had considerable difficulty in convincing them that they were wrong. Finally I persuaded them to do the best they could and see just what happened in a month's time. After a good deal of persuasion I was able to get them to do their best, and the results in a month's time were more than gratifying.

"I remember in one city I had quite a number of old people in one of my classes. With this particular Rite–Number Four–they could just barely get their bodies off the floor; they couldn't get it anywhere near a horizontal position. In the same class were several much younger persons who had no difficulty in performing the Rite perfectly from the very start. This so discouraged the older people that I had to ask the younger ones to refrain from practicing it before their older classmates. I explained that I could not do it at first, either; that I couldn't do a bit better than any of them; but that I could perform the Rite 50 times in succession now without feeling the slightest strain on nerves or muscles; and in order to convince them, I did it right before their eyes. From then on, the class broke all records for results accomplished.

"The only difference between youth and virility, and old age and senility, is simply the difference in the rate of speed at which the Vortexes are spinning. Normalize the different speeds, and the old man becomes a new man again."

Rite Number Five

"The best way to perform this Rite is to place the hands on the floor about two feet apart. Then, with the legs stretched out to the rear with the feet also about two feet apart, push the body, and especially the hips, up as far as possible, rising on the toes and hands. At the same time the head should be brought so far down that the chin comes up against the chest.

"Next, allow the body to come slowly down to a 'sagging' position. Bring the head up, causing it to be drawn as far back as possible.

"After a few weeks, that is after you become quite proficient in this movement, let the body drop from its highest position to a point almost but not quite touching the floor. The muscles should be tensed for a moment when the body is at the highest point, and again at the lowest point. Before the end of the first week this particular Rite will be one of the easiest ones to perform for the average person.

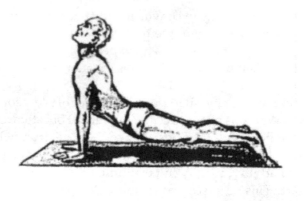

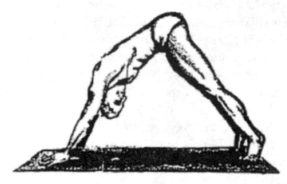

RITE No. 5

"Everywhere I go," went on the Colonel, "folks, at first, call these Rites physical culture exercises. I would like to make it clearly understood that these are not physical culture exercises at all. They are only performed a few times a day; so few times that they could not possibly be of any value as physical culture movements. What the Rites actually do is this: They start the seven Vortexes spinning at a normal rate of speed; at the speed which is normal for, say, a young, strong, robust, virile man of twenty five years of age.

"Now in such a person the Vortexes are all spinning normally at the same rate of speed. On the other hand, if you could view the seven Vortexes of the average middle-aged man—weak, unhealthy, and semi-virile, as he is—you would notice at once that some of the Vortexes had greatly slowed down in their spinning movement; and worse still, all were spinning at a different rate of speed—none of them working together in harmony. The slower ones allowed that part of the body which they govern to degenerate, deteriorate, and become diseased. The faster ones, spinning at a much greater speed, would have caused nervousness and nerve exhaustion. All of them making the individual anything but a real man.

"The only INNER difference between youth and senility, is simply the difference in the rate of speed at which the Vortexes are spinning. Normalize the different speeds, and the old man becomes a new man again."

Further Information

When the Colonel had finished his description of the Five Rites, I said to him, "Let me ask you some questions now."

"Very well," he replied. "That is just what I want you to do."

"I feel that from your description I understand the Rites quite well," I began, "but when and how often are they to be employed?"

"They can be used either night and morning," answered the Colonel, "in the morning only, or just at night, if it is more convenient. I use them both morning and night, but I would not advise so much stimulation for the beginner until he has practiced them for about four months. At the start he could use them the full number of times in the morning, and then in the evening he could gradually build up until finally he is doing the same amount of practice as in the morning."

"Just how many times a day should a man use these Rites?" was my next question.

"To start with," said he, "I would suggest you practice each Rite three times a day for the first week. Then increase them by two a day each week until you are doing 21 a day; which will be at the beginning of the 10th week. If you cannot practice Rite Number One, the whirling one, the same number of times as the others, then do it only as many times as you can without getting too dizzy. The time will come, however, when you can practice it the full number of 21 times.

"I knew of one man who required more than a year before he could do it that many times. But he performed the other four without difficulty, gradually increasing the number until he was doing the full 21 on all four. He got very splendid results.

"Under certain conditions," added the Colonel, "there are some who find it difficult to perform Rite Number One at all, to begin with. But after having done the other four for about six months they are amazed at how easy it is to do Number One. Likewise with the other Rites. If for any reason one or more of them cannot be used, do not be discouraged; use what you can. Results, in that case, will be a little slower, but that is the only handicap.

"If one has been recently operated on for, say, appendicitis, or is afflicted with hernia, he should be very cautious in practicing Rites Number Two and Five. If one is very heavy, he should be cautious in the use of Number Five until his weight has been greatly reduced.

"All five of the Rites are of importance. Even though he may not be able to perform them the prescribed number of times, the individual may rest assured that just a few times each day will be of benefit.

"If, at the end of the fourth week, one finds that he cannot perform every one of the Rites the required number of times, he should note carefully the ones which he is forced to slight. Then, if he is performing the Five Rites in the morning, he should try to make up the deficiency in the evening. Or if he is performing the Rites in the evening, he should endeavor to find time in the morning to catch up. In either event he should not neglect the other Rites, and above all he should never strain himself. If he goes about performing the Rites in an easy, interesting manner it will not be long before he finds everything working out satisfactorily, and that he is doing the Rites the required 21 times a day.

"Some people, acting on their own initiative, invent little aids for their practices. An old fellow in India found it impossible for him to perform Rite Number Four properly even once. He wouldn't be satisfied with just getting his body off the floor; he was determined that it should reach a horizontal position as the Rite prescribed. So he got a box about ten inches high and two and a half feet long. Upon this he put some bedding folded to the right size, and across this padded box he lay flat on his back. Then, with his feet on the floor at one end and his hands on the floor at the other he found it quite simple to raise his body to a horizontal position.

"Now while this little 'stunt' may not in itself have helped the old gentleman in performing the Rite the full 21 times, still the psychological effect of being able to raise his body as high as the much stronger men was undoubtedly quite stimulating and may have been quite beneficial. I do not particularly recommend this old man's aid, although it may help those who think it impossible to make progress in any other way; but if you have an inventive mind you will think of ways and means to help you in performing the more difficult Rites.

"These Rites are so powerful that if one were left out entirely while the other four were practiced regularly the full number of times, only the finest kind of results would be experienced. Only one Rite alone will do wonders as evidenced by the Whirling Dervishes of whom we spoke. Had they spun around only a limited number of times, they would have found themselves greatly benefited, although they may not have attributed their improved condition to the whirling. The fact that they whirled from left to right and that the old men, who no doubt whirled around less than the younger ones, were virile and strong is ample proof that just one Rite will have powerful effects. So if any one finds that they simply cannot perform all five of these practices or that they cannot perform them all the full number of times, they may still know that good results will be experienced from what they are able to do."

"Does anything else go with these Five Rites?" I asked. "There are two more things which would help. The first is to stand erect with hands on hips between the Five Rites and take one or two deep breaths. The other suggestion is to take either a tepid bath or a cool, but not cold, one after practicing the Rites. Going over the body quickly with a wet towel and then with a dry one is probably even better. One thing I must caution you against: you must never take a shower, tub, or wet towel bath which is cold enough to chill you even slightly internally. If you do, you will have undone all the good you have gained from performing the Five Rites."

"This all seems so simple," I ventured, "do you mean to tell me that this is all that is necessary in the work of restoring senile, old men to robust health, vigor, and virility?"

"All that is required," answered the Colonel, "is to practice the Five Rites three times a day to begin with, and gradually increase them as I have explained until each is being practiced 21 times each day. That is all; there is nothing more.

"Of course," he continued, "one must practice them every day in order to keep one's robust vitality. You may skip one day a week, but never more than that. The use of the Five Rites is no hardship at all; it requires less than 10 minutes a day to practice them. If necessary one can get up ten minutes earlier or go to bed ten minutes later.

"The Five Rites are for the express purpose of restoring a man to manhood. That is, to make him virile and keep him that way constantly. Whether or not he will make the comeback in youthful appearance, as I have done in so short a time, depends on how he uses his virility. Some men do not care whether they look young, or even whether they appear young, just so long as they have all their manly powers. But as for me, I was an old man for so many years, practically forty, that I like the idea of throwing off the years in every way possible."

Part Two

It had been ten weeks since Colonel Bradford's return from India. Much had happened in that time. I had immediately started putting the Five Rites into practice and had been getting most gratifying results. The Colonel had been busy with some personal business transactions and I saw little of him for a while, but when he once more was at leisure, I lost no time telling him of my progress and in enthusiastically expressing my feeling regarding this wonderful new system of regaining health, vigor, power, virility, and vitality.

Ever since the day I was sure that I was well on the way to new youth and vigor, I had been thinking of what a splendid idea it would be to pass on the information about the Five Rites to my friends, and now that the Colonel had time to spare, I approached him with the idea of forming a class. He agreed that it was a very commendable idea and agreed to teach it himself on three conditions.

The first of these conditions was that the class should comprise a cross section of men from all walks of life from ditchdiggers to bankers. The second condition was that no member could be under 50 years of age, although they could be up to a hundred or more, if I knew any one that old. These two conditions met with my satisfaction, but the third was a big disappointment. The Colonel insisted that the class be limited to 15 members, and I had ten times that number in mind. However, no amount of persuasion and coercion could change his mind.

From the beginning, the class was a huge success. We met once a week and my friends all had implicit faith in the Colonel and in the Five Rites. As early as the second week, I could see marked improvement in several of them, although, being forbidden to discuss their progress with anyone but the Colonel, I could not verify my impression. However, at the end of a month, we held a kind of testimonial meeting. Every man reported improvement. Some told most glowing accounts; a few, most remarkable ones. A man nearing 75 years of age had made more gains than any of the others.

The weekly meetings of "The Himalaya Club," as we had named it, continued. The tenth week rolled around and practically all of the members were performing all Five Rites 21 times a day. All of them were feeling better and some claimed to have dropped age from their appearance and jokingly gave their ages as younger than they really were. This brought to mind that several of them had asked the Colonel his age but that he had told them he would wait until the end of the tenth week to tell them. This was the evening, but as yet the Colonel had not put in an appearance. Someone suggested that each member write on a slip of paper what age he believed the Colonel to be and then they would compare notes. As the papers were being collected, in walked Colonel Bradford. When he was told what had taken place he said,

"Bring them to me and I shall see how well you have estimated my age. Then I shall tell you what it really is."

The slips all read from 38 to 42, and with great amusement, the Colonel read them aloud. "Gentlemen," he said, "I thank you. You are most complimentary. And as you have been honest with me, I shall be equally honest with you. I shall be 73 years of age on my next birthday." The members stared in consternation and amazement. They found it hard to believe that one so youthful in appearance could have lived so long. Then they wanted to know why, inasmuch as they already felt half their former age, they, too, had not made more progress in youthful appearance.

"In the first place, gentlemen," the Colonel informed them, "you have only been doing this wonderful work for ten weeks. When you have been at it two years you will see a much more pronounced change. Then again, I have not told you all there is to know. I have given you Five Rites which are for the express purpose of restoring one to manly vigor and vitality.

These Five Rites also make one appear more youthful; but if you really want to look and be young in every respect there is a Sixth Rite that you must practice. I have said nothing about it until now because it would have been useless to you without first having obtained good results from the other five."

The Colonel then informed them that in order to go further with the aid of this Sixth Rite, it would be necessary for them to lead a more or less continent life. He suggested that they take a week to think the matter over and decide whether or not they desired to do so for the rest of their lives. Then those who wished to go on would be given Rite Number Six. There were but five who came back the next week, although according to the Colonel this was a better showing than he had experienced with any of his classes in India.

When he had first told them about the Sixth Rite, the Colonel had made it clear that the procreative energy would be lifted up, and that this lifting-up process would cause not only the mind to be renewed but the entire body as well; but that it entailed certain restrictions with which the average man did not care to conform. Then he went on with this explanation.

"In the average virile man," said the Colonel, "the life forces course downward, but in order to become a Superman they must be turned upward. This we call 'The Newer Use of the Reproductive Energy.' Turning these powerful forces upward is a very simple matter, yet man has attempted it in many ways for centuries and in almost every instance has failed. Whole religious orders in the Occidental World have tried this very thing, but they, too, have failed because they have tried to master the procreative energy by suppressing it. There is only one way to master this powerful urge, and that is not by dissipating or suppressing it but by transmuting it—transmuting it and at the same time lifting it upward. In this way you really and truly have discovered not only the 'Elixir of Life,' as the ancients called it, but you have put it to use as well, which is something the ancients were seldom able to do.

"Now this Rite Number Six is the simplest thing in the world to perform. It should only be practiced when one has an excess of procreative energy; when there is a natural desire for its expression. It can be done so easily that it can be performed anywhere at any time. When one feels the powerful reproductive urge, here is all that is necessary:

"Stand erect and then let all the air out of the lungs, as one bends over and places his hands on his knees. Force out the last trace of air. Then, with empty lungs, stand erect, place hands on hips, and push down on them. This has a tendency to push up the shoulders. While doing this, pull in the abdomen just as far as possible, which raises the chest. Now hold this position as long as you can. Then when you are forced to take air into the empty lungs, let the air flow in through the nose. Exhale it through the mouth as you relax the arms and let them hang naturally at your sides. Then take several deep breaths through the mouth or nose and allow them to quickly escape through either the mouth or the nose. This constitutes one complete performance of Rite Number Six. About three are required to subdue the most masculine urge and to turn the powerful procreative or reproductive forces upward.

"The only difference there is between the average virile man and the Superman is that the virile lets the procreative urge flow downward while the Super-man turns the procreative urge upward and reproduces within himself a NEW MAN—a strong, powerful, magnetic man who is constantly growing younger, day by day, moment by moment. This is the true SUPER-MAN, who creates within himself the true 'ELIXIR OF LIFE.' Now you understand why it was unnecessary for me to have left my native England to find the 'Fountain of Youth'—it was within me all the time. Now you can see that when I wrote my friend here some time ago that I had found 'The Fountain of Youth' and was bringing it back with me, I meant just that. The Five Rites and the 'Fountain' are one.

"When I remember Ponce de Leon and his futile search for the 'Fountain' I think of how simple it would have been for him to stay at home and simply use it; but he, like myself, believed it was anywhere in the world except within one's self.

"Please understand that in order to perform Rite Number Six it is absolutely necessary that a man have full masculine virility. He couldn't possibly raise up and transmute procreative energy if there were little or none to transmute. It is absolutely impossible for the impotent man or the one with little virility to perform this Rite. He shouldn't even attempt it, because it would only lead to discouragement, which might do him great harm. Instead he should first practice the other Five Rites until he has full masculine power, and this regardless of how young or how old he may be. Then when the first "full bloom of youth" is experienced within him, he may, if he wishes, go on to the business of being a SUPER-MAN.

"The man of the world is interested only in the material things of the world, and for that reason should practice only the first five Rites until he feels the urge or desire within to become the SUPER-MAN. Then he should decide definitely; for a clean-cut start and a new life are absolutely necessary to those who lead the SUPER-LIFE. They are the ones who become MYSTICS, OCCULTISTS, and ADEPTS. They it is who truly see with THE EYE OF REVELATION."

"Again I say, let no man concern himself with the up-turning of the sex currents until he is thoroughly satisfied in his own mind and heart that he truly desires to lead the life of the MYSTIC; then let him make the step forward, and success will crown his every effort."

Part Three

After the tenth week, Colonel Bradford no longer attended each weekly meeting. However, he still kept up his interest in the "Himalaya Club," and from time to time would speak on various subjects which would aid them in their work. Sometimes the members requested him to advise them on some particular subject. For instance, we discussed among ourselves one night the tremendously important part that food played in our lives. How the right food would make us more alive and vigorous while the wrong food would make us sluggish and dull. None of us knew much about the subject, however, so we requested the Colonel to advise us at our next meeting as to the Lamas' policy regarding food.

"In the Himalayan Lamasery where I was a neophyte," said the Colonel, in addressing us the following week, "there are no problems concerning the right foods, nor in getting sufficient food. Each of the Lamas does his share of the work in producing what is needed. Furthermore, all the work is done by the most primitive means. Even the soil is spaded by hand. Of course, the Lamas could use horses and plows if they so desired, but direct contact with the soil, handling it and working with it, seems to add something to man's existence. Personally, it made me feel very strongly that I was a part of the Universal. Not merely working with it or working for it but rather that the Universal and I were one.

"Now it is true that the Lamas are vegetarians, but not strictly so. They do use eggs, butter, and cheese in quantities sufficient to serve certain functions of the brain, body, and nervous system. But aside from this they do not need meat, for all who are strong and virile, and who practice Rite Number Six have no need of meat, fish, or fowl.

"Most of those who join the ranks of the Lamas are men of the world who know little about proper food and diet. Yet they are only in the Grand Retreat in the Himalayas a very short while when they begin to show wonderful signs of physical improvement, due no doubt to the diet in the Lamasery.

"No Lama is choosy about his meals. He can't be because there is little to choose from. A Lama diet consists of good, wholesome food but as a rule it consists of but one article of food to a meal that in itself is a secret of health. When one eats just one kind of food at a time there can be no clashing of foods in the stomach. Foods clash in the stomach because starches will not mix with proteins. For example, bread, which is starchy, when eaten with meats, eggs, or cheese, which are protein, sets up a reaction in the stomach which often causes not only immediate physical pain, but which contributes as well to a short life and a not particularly merry one.

"Many times in the Lamasery dining hall I have set down to the table along with the Lamas and eaten a meal consisting solely of bread. At other times I have had nothing but fresh vegetables and fresh fruits, while at still another meal I ate nothing but cooked vegetables and cooked fruits. At first I greatly missed the large variety of foods to which I had been accustomed; but after a short while I could eat and enjoy a meal consisting of nothing but dark bread or some one particular fruit. Sometimes it would be a feast of one vegetable.

"The point I wish to bring out to you gentlemen is not that you should resign yourselves to a diet of one kind of food to a meal but that you should keep starches, fruits, and vegetables separate from meats, fish, and fowl at your meals.

"It is permissible to make a meal of just meat. In fact, you could have several kinds of meats to a meal. You can have butter, eggs, and cheese with the meat meal, and dark bread, and, if you wish, coffee, or tea, but you must not end up with anything sweet or starchy. No pies or cakes or puddings.

"Then again, your meal can be strictly starches. Then you can indulge in all the sweet fruits, all the bread, butter, pies, cakes, puddings, and fresh or cooked vegetables you like without feeling any ill effects. But keep these meals separate.

"Butter seems to be a neutral. It can be used with either a starchy meal or with a meat meal. Milk, however, agrees better with starch meals. Coffee and tea should always be taken black, never with cream, although a small amount of sweetening will do no harm.

"The proper use of eggs was another interesting and beneficial thing that came to my attention while dwelling in the Lamasery. The Lamas would not eat whole eggs unless they were engaged in hard manual labor; then they might eat one, medium-boiled. However, they did indulge to a very great extent in raw egg, discarding the white part. Before I learned better it seemed a waste of perfectly good food to throw the cooked whites to the chickens, but now I know that no one should eat the whites of eggs unless he is doing hard manual labor; the egg whites are used only by the muscles.

"Although I had always been aware of the fact that egg yolks were particularly good for one, it wasn't until after I arrived at the Lamasery and had an opportunity to talk with an old Austrian chemist that I learned their true value. Then I was amazed to find out that just common hen eggs contain at least half of the sixteen elements required by the brain, nerves, blood, and tissues. It is true that these elements are only needed in small quantities, but they must be included in the diet if one is to be exceptionally robust and healthy, both mentally and physically.

"There is one thing more of great importance that I learned from the Lamas. They taught me to eat, not slowly for its own sake, but so that I might masticate my food more thoroughly. Their bread is tough and it takes good chewing to reduce it to a liquid before swallowing it, but this I learned to do.

"Everything one eats should be 'digested,' so to speak, in the mouth before allowing it to enter the stomach. Starches, particularly, must be digested in the mouth. Unless they first are thoroughly mixed with saliva they literally are dynamite when they get to the stomach.

"While one can do with little mastication of protein foods, such as meat, fish, and fowl, it is a sensible thing to chew them well anyhow. More nourishment can be obtained from food when it is thoroughly masticated. This necessitates less food, and often the amount can be reduced by one-half.

"Many things which I had casually taken for granted before entering the Lamasery seemed shocking when I left it two years later. One of the first things I noted upon arriving in one of the larger cities in India was the prodigious amount of food consumed by everyone who could afford to do so. I have seen one man eat a quantity of food at a meal sufficient to feed four hard-working Lamas and keep them alive and thriving. Providing, of course, that the Lamas would put that variety of food in their stomachs, which they would not do.

"Variety was another thing which appalled me. Having been in the habit of eating but one or two foods at a meal, it amazed me to count

23 varieties of food one evening on my host's table. No wonder that the English and the Americans have such miserable stomachs and such damnably poor health. They seem to know nothing whatsoever about the kind of food they should eat for health and strength.

"Just the other evening I had dinner with a very learned man. He was an educator and quite an intellectual. He calmly stated, while we waited to be served, that in a few short years the human race could become really worthwhile providing his ideas were thoroughly carried out. This man was an excellent dictator type, and I was quite impressed by his knowledge, his original ideas, and his ability to express himself. But when I saw this man's selection of food at the dinner table, my opinion of him changed. It was the most atrocious combination of nutritive TNT I ever saw. I thought, if I could only give him some simple ideas about food he could become a really worthwhile force for good in the world in a few short weeks.

"The right food, the right combinations of foods, the right amount of food, and the right method of eating food combines to do great things for one. It will enable one to put on weight if he is underweight, and to reduce if he is overweight. There are many other things of a different character that I should like to tell you tonight, but we haven't time. Keep in mind these five things:

1. "Never eat starch and meat at the same meal; although if you are strong and healthy it need not cause you too much concern now.
2. "If coffee bothers you, drink it black, using no milk or cream. If it bothers you then, discontinue its use.
3. "Chew your food to a liquid and cut down on the amount as much as possible.
4. "By all means and before all else eat raw egg yolks once a day, every day. Take them at meal times but not with the meals; rather just before or just after.
5. "Reduce the varieties of food to a minimum. If one is really hungry before he starts eating, the tendency to desire many different foods is lost in hunger."

Part Four

Colonel Bradford was speaking before the "Himalaya Club" for the last time before leaving on a tour of the United States and a visit to his native England. He had selected for his subject the things that help youthify a man, regardless of whether or not he practices Rite Number Six. As the Colonel spoke, he seemed to be keener, more alert and vigorous, and virile than ever before. Upon his return from the Lamasery, he had struck me as the acme of perfection; yet since then he had kept right on improving, and even now was making new gains constantly.

"There are several things I want to talk about tonight," began the Colonel, "which I am sure will interest you. The first of them is the human voice. Do you realize that when one has made a study of men's voices he can tell instantly how much masculine vitality a man possesses just by hearing him speak? You have all heard the shrill, piping voice of an old man. Well, when a man's voice begins to take on that high pitch he is in a very deplorable condition. Let me explain.

"The Vortex at the base of the neck has power over the vocal cords. This Vortex and the one below in the sex center are directly connected. Of course, all the Vortexes have a common connection, but these two are geared together, as it were. What affects one affects the other, so that when a man's voice is high his manly vitality is low.

"Now all that is necessary to speed up these two Vortexes, along with the others, is to practice the Five Rites. However, one does not have to wait until these Vortexes are increased in speed by the use of the Five Rites, but can raise their speed of vibration with a special method that works very well. This particular practice is easy. It consists in simply putting forth an effort to keep the voice low; not allowing it to become high, shrill, or piping. Listen to men with good low voices and become conscious of how a real man's voice sounds. Then whenever you talk, keep the voice down to the masculine pitch as much as possible.

"Real old men will find this to be quite a little task; but it brings results. The first thing you know the lowered voice will speed up the Vortex in the base of the throat. That will speed up the Vortex in the sex center, which will improve the man in masculine energy, and this again will cause the Vortex in the throat to speed up. The adolescent boy whose voice is changing is experiencing the same thing. The Two Vortexes are speeding up. In this case it is usually caused by the Vortex in the procreative center being speeded up by nature. But anything that will speed up the Vortex in the throat will cause its companion Vortex immediately below to increase speed.

"There are a number of young men who are robust and virile now who will not remain that way long. This is due to the fact that their particular voice, for several reasons which I haven't the time to explain now, never came down to the masculine pitch. But these young men, as well as the old ones, can definitely get results of a very wonderful nature by consciously lowering their voices. In the young men it will mean prolonged virility; in the older men, renewed virility.

"Some time ago I came across a quite splendid voice exercise. Like all other potent things it is very simple. Whenever you are by yourself or where there is sufficient noise to drown your voice so that you will not annoy others, practice saying in low masculine voice, partly through the nose:

"Me—me–me–me-me

"Repeat it time and again. When you get it down quite low, try it in a small room, like the bathroom. You can often make the room hum with your voice. Then try to get the same effect in a larger room. Of course, listening to this vibration of your voice is not entirely necessary; but often the vibration will cause the other Vortexes in the body to speed up, especially the one in the sex center and the two in the head.

"I might add that in old women, the voice also becomes shrill and should be toned down. Of course, a woman's voice naturally is higher than a man's. If she should get it down as low as a man's, it would not be beneficial at all to her. It would speed up the Two Vortexes—the one in the throat and its companion, so as to cause her to act, look, think, and talk mannishly. By the same token, a mannish woman could wonderfully improve herself by raising her voice to the level of a normal woman's.

"I have known of men with high voices who partook of so much alcoholic beverages that they developed 'whiskey' voices–low and growling. To their amazement they began to become virile again. Usually they attributed their good fortune to intemperance or to a certain brand of whiskey, but neither intemperance nor whiskey did anything for them directly. What happened was that the vocal cords were irritated and therefore inflamed and swollen. This lowered the voice and raised the speed of the Vortex in the throat, which in turn, raised the vibrations of the Vortex in the masculine center below, and brought about the renewed masculine vitality.

"Now," said the Colonel, after pausing a moment, "I want to speak on one more subject, which could be entitled 'Putting off the old man.'

Lowering the voice and speeding up the Vortexes certainly has a lot to do in eliminating the 'old man' within us, but there are other things which help to make us much younger even though they do not directly affect the Vortexes. If it were possible suddenly to take a man out of a decrepit old body and place him in a brand new youthful one about 25 years of age, I am confident that the old man he had allowed himself to become would cause him to remain old in most of his ways. It is true that he would perk up a bit around the ladies, but outside of that I think he would remain old.

"Getting old, of course, is brought about first by a lack or a complete absence of manly virility. But that is not the only cause. The world is full of old men around 60 who get a certain dubious pleasure out of acting old. This is all wrong. Regardless of whether a man has full vitality at the present time or not, he should do everything possible to eliminate the 'old man' that has crept within him. He must be dislodged and rooted out. Therefore, gentlemen, from now on get rid of the 'old man' within you. How to do it? It is very simple. Don't do the things old people do. With your new and ever-increasing vitality this should be easy.

"The first thing to do is to straighten up. Stand like a man should. When you first started this class, some of you were so bent over that you looked like question marks; but as vigor returned and spirits became better you began to straighten up. That was fine; but don't stop now. Straighten right on up, start throwing your chest out, pull the stomach and the chin in, and right away you have eliminated 20 years from your appearance and 40 years from your mind.

"Then eliminate 'old man' mannerisms. When you walk, know first where you are going; then start out and go there. Don't dog-trot or run, and don't shuffle along, but pick up your feet and stride. Keep one eye on where you are going and the other one on everything you pass.

"At the Himalayan Lamasery there was a man, a European, whom you would have sworn was not over 35 years of age, and who acted like a man of 25 in every respect. This man was over a hundred, and if I told you how much over a hundred you would not believe me.

"Now about your weight. If you are underweight, you can throw off the years by increasing your weight. If you are overweight, which is a splendid sign of old age and senility, you can throw off more years by reducing the weight to normal. Get rid of the enlarged abdomens, too, and you will look 10 years younger immediately.

Method

trenuous method of awakening
ed in the chapters above may be
especially those with health or
ticed by anyone. Begin with all
n to the second stage when this
rd stage when the second stage
ge for at least three years of daily

e One

egin by loosening yo
ght belts and tight b

easy chair, wit
your sides. Br
ess tension t

n, draw in a slow
your diaphragm
s.

r throat, slowly
rd and the belly
roat if you hear
the throat open,
when your lungs

, and then raise
owly each time.
the air in your
aging the solar
ng tissues.

and normally
three times at
ork gradually
ove, each one
ning.

id water—not
ou: tub bath,
as options in

solar plexus.
vely straight
ture or any
o is the seiza
tices, which
then sitting
on posture,
far enough
air, and the
es.

know
ready r
who nee
I must be o
Of course, v
were glad and t
The thought that th
find "The Fountain o
of Life," thrilled us. Tru
upon the world.

- When you have released as much tension as you ca[n] deep breath and push out your belly, drawing dow[n] so that the air goes to the very bottom of your lung[s]. Without breathing out, but without closing you[r] raise the diaphragm so that the chest pushes outw[ard] sinks in. You will know if you have closed your t[hroat] make an effort to breathe a little more air in even [when] a soft "pop" just before you breathe out. To keep [the] are full.

- Still holding the breath, slowly lower the diaphragm[,] it again; lower it again, and raise it again, moving s[lowly] Then lower it one more time. This process moves [the] lungs from the bottom of the lungs to the top, mass[aging] plexus and also cleansing and strengthening your lu[ngs]. Let the breath out slowly and evenly. Breathe deep[ly] for a while, and then repeat. Do the whole sequenc[e] first. When this is easy, add a fourth repetition, and [work] up to twenty repetitions of the pattern described a[bove] separated from the next by a period of ordinary breat[hing].

Washing:

- Wash your entire body once each day with cool or tep[id] hot, and not cold. The method of washing is up to [you] shower, or sponge or washcloth bath are all mentioned [in] the sources and seem to be equally effective.

Solar Plexus Concentration:

- Spend five minutes each day concentrating on your To do this, sit in any position that leaves your spine relat[ively] and supported only by your own muscles. Lotus other standard Indian meditation posture is suit[able] posture used in Japanese martial arts and e is done by kneeling with the feet stretche back on your heels. So is the standar sitting in a chair with your feet fla forward that your back does no hands palm down on the thi

- Once you settle into the position, relax all the muscles that you don't need to maintain the position, then turn your attention to your solar plexus and breathe slowly, steadily, and gently while imagining a sphere of pale golden light a few inches across in the solar plexus. See and feel it radiating light all through your body. After the five minutes are up, release the imagery and go about the rest of your day.

Stage Two

Continuation of Basic Practices:

- Continue doing the breathing exercise and daily washing exactly as described above.

Solar Plexus and Pineal Gland Concentration:

- Do the solar plexus concentration for five minutes exactly as described above. Then draw in a breath and imagine a current of light rising up the midline of your body from your solar plexus to a point inside your head halfway between the upper parts of your two ears. As you breathe out, imagine the point radiating a gentle, steady light, which may be of any color that comes naturally to you. Let the light fill the back of your head. Do this three times with three breaths in sequence.

Stage Three

- Continue all the practices of the second stage exactly as given above. The following steps are added to the solar plexus and pineal gland concentration exercise, just after the completion of the steps listed above.
- Using both hands, gently massage the back of the head and neck for a minute or so.
- Concentrate again on the pineal gland center. Imagine it as a radiant star filling the back of your head with its light. The light may be of any color that occurs to you naturally.
- Imagine the light flowing down your spinal column all the way to the base of your spine, then over to your left leg, and all the wa

down to the sole of your left foot. Imagine the light pooling there, as though it is filling your leg up from the bottom of your sole. As the light fills your foot, tense every muscle in your foot; as it fills your lower leg, tense every muscle there; as it fills your thigh, tense every muscle there, until your entire left leg from hip to toes is tensed and full of light.

- Do exactly the same thing with the right leg, sending a current of light from your pineal gland down your spine to the base and then over and down to the sole of your right foot, tensing your right leg a little at a time as it fills with light. Keep your left leg tense as you do this.

- Do the same thing to your torso from the base up to the level of the armpits, filling it with light and tensing the muscles. Then send the current of light down your left arm to the fingertips, filling the arm a little at a time with light and tensing the muscles. Then do the same thing with your right arm. Finally, bring the light up to fill your shoulders, your neck, and your head and face, tensing these as well. By the time the light reaches the crown of your head, your entire body should be tense from top to bottom.

- Relax the tensions in the order you established them, beginning with the left foot and leg, then the right foot and leg, then the torso to the armpits, and so on. As you relax them, keep the awareness of the light filling your body. As you end this phase, your muscles are relaxed and your whole body is full of the light that radiated from your pineal gland. This completes the practice; take a few ordinary breaths and then go about the rest of your day.

Additional Practices

- Consider doing the Rising Call exercise given above on pages 17–18. It should be done only once a day, at a different time than the other exercises just given.
- Consider adding the Carey protocol, which is given in Appendix 2 on pages 139–144.

The Carey Protocol

While George W. Carey's cell salt protocol is not strictly speaking part of the system of spiritual alchemy that unfolds from the Five Rites, it is a closely related system that aims at the same goal using means that are completely compatible with the inner alchemy this book has explored. That compatibility is not simply a matter of theory: I have experimented with combining the two systems, and the results have been good. For this reason, I have included a complete explanation of Carey's protocol below, for readers who may be interested in putting it to work by itself or in conjunction with the Five Rites and concentration on the vortices.

The first step in the Carey protocol is determining the location of the sun at the date and time when you were born. If you have cast your own horoscope, you can find that information on it; if not, there are dozens of online websites that will calculate a free horoscope for you. If you don't know your exact time of birth, that doesn't matter for this purpose. As seen from earth, the sun moves through the heavens at a rate of one degree every day, and to use the protocol it is enough to know the sun's position within a ten-degree window.

Once you know the position of your natal sun, look it up on the following table.

Natal Sun	Cell Salts
11°0′–20°59′	Calc. Sulph. 1, Silicea 3, Calc. Phos. 3, Nat. Mur. 2
21°0′–30°	Silicea 3, Calc. Phos. 3, Nat. Mur. 3
0°0′–10°59′ Sagittarius	Silicea 2, Calc. Phos. 3, Nat. Mur. 3, Fer Phos. 1
11°0′–20°59′	Silicea 1, Calc. Phos. 3, Nat. Mur. 3, Phos. 2
21°0′–30°	Calc. Phos. 3, Nat. Mur. 3, Ferru
0°0′–10°59′ Capricorn	Calc. Phos. 2, Nat. Mur. 3, Ferr Kali Phos. 1
11°0′–20°59′	Calc. Phos. 1, Nat. Mur. 3, F Kali Phos. 2
21°0′–30°	Nat. Mur. 3, Ferrum Ph
0°0′–10°59′ Aquarius	Nat. Mur. 2, Ferrum P Nat. Sulph. 1
11°0′–20°59′	Nat. Mur. 1, Ferrur Nat. Sulph. 2
21°0′–30°	Ferrum Phos. 3,
0°0′–10°59′ Pisces	Ferrum Phos.
11°0′–20°59′	Kali Mur. 1
11°0′–20°59′	Ferrum Ph Kali Mur
21°0′–30°59′	Kali Pho

the cryptic-looking indications
w many doses of which cell
reviations for the cell salt
pose (and for the purpo
t homeopathic supply
he 6x potency: that
m.[1] Cell salts car
your body all th
(milk sugar). I′
products, the
athic suppl

dilution

The numbers following each abbreviation indicate how many tablets to take in each dose. If your natal sun was at 5° Aries, in other words, each dose consists of two tablets of Kali Phos. 6x, three tablets of Nat. Sulph. 6x, three tablets of Kali Mur. 6x, and one tablet of Calc. Fluor. 6x; nine tablets in all. These are placed under the tongue and allowed to dissolve. If you prefer to take cell salts in liquid form, use as many drops of each cell salt as you would use tablets, put them in a half glass of water, and drink it down.

The next point is of crucial importance. You take three of these doses each month when the moon is in the same sign as your natal sun. If the sun was in Aries when you were born, in other words, you take three doses of the cell salts listed in the table during the time when the moon is in Aries each month. The moon takes two to two and a half days to pass through each sign of the zodiac. Following on the example above, if your natal sun was at 5° Aries, each month you would take the dose of nine tablets listed above three times while the moon is in Aries. Try to space the doses more or less equally: for example, if the moon enters Aries early one morning and leaves it in the afternoon two and a half days later, take one dose the first morning, the second dose the second morning, and the third the third morning before the moon passes into Taurus.

How can you tell when the moon is in Aries? These days there is an abundance of websites, computer programs, and phone apps that will track the moon through the zodiac for you. If you prefer to do things in a somewhat more low-tech way, any astrological calendar or ephemeris will give you the times and days when the moon enters each sign, and so will most old-fashioned almanacs. Remember that the moon does the rounds of the zodiac in a little less than a month, so that now and then there will be a month where you will be taking your cell salts twice, once for a few days at the beginning of the month and once for a few days at the end.

Premature or Postmature Birth

Please note that all this assumes that you were born after nine months in your mother's womb in the usual way. If you were a premature baby, you will need to add additional cell salts to the mix. The rule here is simple: take the position of the sun at your actual birth date and the position of the sun on the date when you would have been born

"Here is something else which should interest all of you. Only two years ago I was as bald as the baldest man here. When vitality started coming back, one of the Lamas told me to massage my scalp good with a piece of butter twice a week. The butter up there was fresh, not a bit of salt in it. I took his advice and massaged my scalp with butter until it soon loosened up. I did this about one hour after a meal. The food elements in the blood were brought to the scalp by the circulation of the blood. The scalp was so thoroughly massaged that the blood vessels were dilated; the hair roots picked up the necessary nutrition, and the hair grew—as you can plainly see.

"Even though you may not care to become mystics at this time, you can throw many years off your mind, your attitude, and feelings. So start at once. Any effort you put forth will be rewarded, I can assure you. I have given you nothing but simple Rites and practices because the simple things will bring you health, youth, virility, and success when nothing else will.

"It has been a most thrilling thing to see you men change and improve from day to day," concluded the Colonel, "but now you know all there is need for you to know for the present. When you are ready for more information, the teacher will appear. There are others who need this information much more than you gentlemen did and I must be on my way to them."

Of course, we were sorry to see our friend the Colonel depart. But we were glad and thankful for the priceless information he had given us. The thought that the Colonel was soon to help other men like ourselves find "The Fountain of Youth," "The Philosopher's Stone," "The Elixir of Life," thrilled us. Truly, I thought to myself. The Eye of Revelation is upon the world.

The Simplified Method

The older and less physically strenuous method of awakening the Eye of Revelation discussed in the chapters above may be better suited to some people, especially those with health or mobility problems. It may be practiced by anyone. Begin with all three parts of the first stage, go on to the second stage when this comes easily, and go on to the third stage when the second stage comes easily. Maintain the third stage for at least three years of daily practice.

Stage One

Solar Plexus Breathing Exercise:

- This is done once each day. Begin by loosening your clothing so that you can breathe freely; tight belts and tight bras are especially to be avoided.
- Relax on a bed, couch, or easy chair, with legs stretched out and uncrossed, and arms by your sides. Breathe slowly, deeply, and comfortably, and allow all excess tension to drain out of your body.

- When you have released as much tension as you can, draw in a slow deep breath and push out your belly, drawing down your diaphragm so that the air goes to the very bottom of your lungs.
- Without breathing out, but without closing your throat, slowly raise the diaphragm so that the chest pushes outward and the belly sinks in. You will know if you have closed your throat if you hear a soft "pop" just before you breathe out. To keep the throat open, make an effort to breathe a little more air in even when your lungs are full.
- Still holding the breath, slowly lower the diaphragm, and then raise it again; lower it again, and raise it again, moving slowly each time. Then lower it one more time. This process moves the air in your lungs from the bottom of the lungs to the top, massaging the solar plexus and also cleansing and strengthening your lung tissues.
- Let the breath out slowly and evenly. Breathe deeply and normally for a while, and then repeat. Do the whole sequence three times at first. When this is easy, add a fourth repetition, and work gradually up to twenty repetitions of the pattern described above, each one separated from the next by a period of ordinary breathing.

Washing:

- Wash your entire body once each day with cool or tepid water—not hot, and not cold. The method of washing is up to you: tub bath, shower, or sponge or washcloth bath are all mentioned as options in the sources and seem to be equally effective.

Solar Plexus Concentration:

- Spend five minutes each day concentrating on your solar plexus. To do this, sit in any position that leaves your spine relatively straight and supported only by your own muscles. Lotus posture or any other standard Indian meditation posture is suitable. So is the seiza posture used in Japanese martial arts and esoteric practices, which is done by kneeling with the feet stretched out flat, and then sitting back on your heels. So is the standard Western meditation posture, sitting in a chair with your feet flat on the floor, the seat far enough forward that your back does not touch the back of the chair, and the hands palm down on the thighs a little back from the knees.

- Once you settle into the position, relax all the muscles that you don't need to maintain the position, then turn your attention to your solar plexus and breathe slowly, steadily, and gently while imagining a sphere of pale golden light a few inches across in the solar plexus. See and feel it radiating light all through your body. After the five minutes are up, release the imagery and go about the rest of your day.

Stage Two

Continuation of Basic Practices:

- Continue doing the breathing exercise and daily washing exactly as described above.

Solar Plexus and Pineal Gland Concentration:

- Do the solar plexus concentration for five minutes exactly as described above. Then draw in a breath and imagine a current of light rising up the midline of your body from your solar plexus to a point inside your head halfway between the upper parts of your two ears. As you breathe out, imagine the point radiating a gentle, steady light, which may be of any color that comes naturally to you. Let the light fill the back of your head. Do this three times with three breaths in sequence.

Stage Three

- Continue all the practices of the second stage exactly as given above. The following steps are added to the solar plexus and pineal gland concentration exercise, just after the completion of the steps listed above.
- Using both hands, gently massage the back of the head and neck for a minute or so.
- Concentrate again on the pineal gland center. Imagine it as a radiant star filling the back of your head with its light. The light may be of any color that occurs to you naturally.
- Imagine the light flowing down your spinal column all the way to the base of your spine, then over to your left leg, and all the way

down to the sole of your left foot. Imagine the light pooling there, as though it is filling your leg up from the bottom of your sole. As the light fills your foot, tense every muscle in your foot; as it fills your lower leg, tense every muscle there; as it fills your thigh, tense every muscle there, until your entire left leg from hip to toes is tensed and full of light.

- Do exactly the same thing with the right leg, sending a current of light from your pineal gland down your spine to the base and then over and down to the sole of your right foot, tensing your right leg a little at a time as it fills with light. Keep your left leg tense as you do this.

- Do the same thing to your torso from the base up to the level of the armpits, filling it with light and tensing the muscles. Then send the current of light down your left arm to the fingertips, filling the arm a little at a time with light and tensing the muscles. Then do the same thing with your right arm. Finally, bring the light up to fill your shoulders, your neck, and your head and face, tensing these as well. By the time the light reaches the crown of your head, your entire body should be tense from top to bottom.

- Relax the tensions in the order you established them, beginning with the left foot and leg, then the right foot and leg, then the torso to the armpits, and so on. As you relax them, keep the awareness of the light filling your body. As you end this phase, your muscles are relaxed and your whole body is full of the light that radiated from your pineal gland. This completes the practice; take a few ordinary breaths and then go about the rest of your day.

Additional Practices

- Consider doing the Rising Call exercise given above on pages 17–18. It should be done only once a day, at a different time than the other exercises just given.
- Consider adding the Carey protocol, which is given in Appendix 2 on pages 139–144.

Natal Sun	Cell Salts
0°0′–10°59′ Aries	Kali Phos. 2, Nat. Sulph. 3, Kali Mur. 3, Calc. Fluor. 1
11°0′–20°59′	Kali Phos. 1, Nat. Sulph. 3, Kali Mur. 3, Calc. Fluor. 2
21°0′–30°	Nat. Sulph. 3, Kali Mur. 3, Calc. Fluor. 3
0°0′–10°59′ Taurus	Nat. Sulph. 2, Kali Mur. 3, Calc. Fluor. 3, Mag. Phos. 1
11°0′–20°59′	Nat. Sulph. 1, Kali Mur. 3, Calc. Fluor. 3, Mag. Phos. 2
21°0′–30°	Kali Mur. 3, Calc. Fluor. 3, Mag. Phos. 3
0°0′–10°59′ Gemini	Kali Mur. 2, Calc. Fluor. 3, Mag. Phos. 3, Kali Sulph. 1
11°0′–20°59′	"Kali Mur. 1, Calc. Fluor. 3, Mag. Phos. 3, Kali Sulph. 2
21°0′–30°	Calc. Fluor. 3, Mag. Phos. 3, Kali Sulph. 3
0°0′–10°59′ Cancer	Calc. Fluor. 2, Mag. Phos. 3, Kali Sulph. 3, Nat. Phos. 1
11°0′–20°59′	Calc. Fluor. 1, Mag. Phos. 3, Kali Sulph. 3, Nat. Phos. 2
21°0′–30°	Mag. Phos. 3, Kali Sulph. 3, Nat. Phos. 3
0°0′–10°59′ Leo	Mag. Phos. 2, Kali Sulph. 3, Nat. Phos. 3, Calc. Sulph. 1
11°0′–20°59′	Mag. Phos. 1, Kali Sulph. 3, Nat. Phos. 3, Calc. Sulph. 2
21°0′–30°	Kali Sulph. 3, Nat. Phos. 3, Calc. Sulph. 3
0°0′–10°59′ Virgo	Kali Sulph. 2, Nat. Phos. 3, Calc. Sulph. 3, Silicea 1
11°0′–20°59′	Kali Sulph. 1, Nat. Phos. 3, Calc. Sulph. 3, Silicea 2
21°0′–30°	Nat. Phos. 3, Calc. Sulph. 3, Silicea 3
0°0′–10°59′ Libra	Nat. Phos. 2, Calc. Sulph. 3, Silicea 3, Calc. Phos. 1
11°0′–20°59′	Nat. Phos. 1, Calc. Sulph. 3, Silicea 3, Calc. Phos. 2
21°0′–30°	Calc. Sulph. 3, Silicea 3, Calc. Phos. 3
0°0′–10°59′ Scorpio	Calc. Sulph. 2, Silicea 3, Calc. Phos. 3, Nat. Mur. 1

APPENDIX 2

The Carey Protocol

While George W. Carey's cell salt protocol is not strictly speaking part of the system of spiritual alchemy that unfolds from the Five Rites, it is a closely related system that aims at the same goal using means that are completely compatible with the inner alchemy this book has explored. That compatibility is not simply a matter of theory: I have experimented with combining the two systems, and the results have been good. For this reason, I have included a complete explanation of Carey's protocol below, for readers who may be interested in putting it to work by itself or in conjunction with the Five Rites and concentration on the vortices.

The first step in the Carey protocol is determining the location of the sun at the date and time when you were born. If you have cast your own horoscope, you can find that information on it; if not, there are dozens of online websites that will calculate a free horoscope for you. If you don't know your exact time of birth, that doesn't matter for this purpose. As seen from earth, the sun moves through the heavens at a rate of one degree every day, and to use the protocol it is enough to know the sun's position within a ten-degree window.

Once you know the position of your natal sun, look it up on the following table.

Look those up on the table above, and write down the names of all the cell salts listed for those dates and the dates in between. Then write down the highest number of tablets listed with each cell salt, and that gives you the formula for your monthly dose.

For example, let's say you were born when the Sun was at 5° Aries but you were a month premature, so you would have been born at 5° Taurus if things had gone in the normal manner. Look at the table for these sun positions and the ones between.

0°0′–10°59′ Aries	Kali Phos. 2, Nat. Sulph. 3, Kali Mur. 3, Calc. Fluor. 1
11°0′–20°59′	Kali Phos. 1, Nat. Sulph. 3, Kali Mur. 3, Calc. Fluor. 2
21°0′–30°	Nat. Sulph. 3, Kali Mur. 3, Calc. Fluor. 3
0°0′–10°59′ Taurus	Nat. Sulph. 2, Kali Mur. 3, Calc. Fluor. 3, Mag. Phos. 1

The cell salts listed here are Kali Phos., Nat. Sulph., Kali Mur., Calc. Fluor., and Mag. Phos. The highest number listed for Kali Phos. is 2, the highest number for the next three salts is 3, and the only number given with Mag. Phos. is 1. So the dose that you take when the Moon is in Aries, is Kali Phos. 2, Nat. Sulph. 3, Kali Mur. 3, Calc. Fluor. 3, and Mag. Phos. 1.

If you were born after more than nine months in the womb, reduce the cell salts accordingly. Let's say that you were expected when the Sun was at 5° Aries but weren't born until two weeks later when the Sun was at 15°. Here you list the cell salts listed for the dates in question but take the lower number of tablets. If you take the doses listed in the first two lines of the section of the table above, the cell salts listed are Kali Phos., Nat. Sulph., Kali Mur., and Calc. Fluor. The lowest number given for Kali Phos. and Calc Fluor are 1 each, and the other two are listed as 3 each. Your dose when the Moon is in Aries will be Kali Phos. 1, Nat. Sulph. 3, Kali Mur. 3, and Calc. Fluor. 1.

Bioplasma

The one further element of the protocol is a daily dose of Bioplasma, a mixture of the twelve cell salts in the proportions in which they are found in the human body. Bioplasma was invented by George W. Carey, and it is used by many homeopaths today as a general health tonic and as a treatment for athletes. You can purchase Bioplasma from the same homeopathic supply houses that sell cell salts. Put six tablets under the tongue first thing in the morning every day, whether or not you are taking the special cell salt dose given in the table above.

The cell salts and Bioplasma can both be purchased from many shops online, and some food coops and health food stores also carry them. If you aren't sure where to find them, a little searching online will bring up plenty of sources.

If you are interested in learning more about the cell salts and biochemic medicine, the books by Boericke and Dewey, Chapman and Perry, and Weintraub listed in the bibliography are good sources, and the first two are long since out of copyright and can be downloaded free of charge from online archives. George W. Carey's books are also worth studying, but they can be a wild ride for beginners.

Bibliography

Peter Kelder's Text

Only two copies of the original 1939 edition are known to exist, and only one copy of the 1946 edition has apparently survived. I have not been able to consult either of them directly. I used the following editions in my research.

Kelder, Peter, *The Eye of Revelation* (Bayside, CA: Borderland Sciences Research Foundation, 1975). This photostatic reproduction of the 1939 edition was the basis for the text included in this book.

Kelder, Peter, *Ancient Secret of the Fountain of Youth* (Gig Harbor, WA: Harbor Press, 1985). This version underwent considerable revision and refers to the seven spinal chakras instead of the seven vortices given in the original.

Kelder, Peter, *The Eye of Revelation: Ancient Anti-Aging Secrets of the Five Tibetan Rites*, ed. Carolinda Witt (Avalon, NSW, Australia: UnMind, 2008). The best of the modern versions, this includes the extra chapters Kelder added to the 1946 edition.

Other Source Material

Arundale, G.S., *Kundalini: An Occult Experience* (Madras: Theosophical Publishing House, 1938)

Atkinson, William Walker. *See* Dumont, Theron Q; Ramacharaka, Yogi.

Avalon, Arthur, *The Serpent Power* (Madras: Ganesh & Co, 1950).

Bedell, Leila G, *The Abdominal Brain* (Chicago, IL: Gross & Delabridge, 1885).

Blavatsky, Helena P., *Esoteric Section Instructions* (London: privately printed, 1889).

Boericke, William, and W.A. Dewey, *The Twelve Tissue Remedies of Schussler* (St. Louis, MO: Luyties, 1914).

Carey, George W., and Inez Eudora Perry, *God-Man: The Word Made Flesh* (Los Angeles, CA: Chemistry of Life, 1920).

Chapman, J.B., and Edward L. Perry, *Biochemic Theory and Practice* (St. Louis, MO: Luyties, 1920).

Cosmic Convergence Research Group, The Back Story to Christian Rosenkreutz and Steiner's "Circle of 12," *Cosmic Convergence* (cosmi-convergence.com/2017/01/26/the-back-story-to-christian-rosen-kreuz-and-steiners-circle-of-12/; downloaded 2/5/2022).

Crowley, Aleister, *Eight Lectures on Yoga* (London: Ordo Templi Orientis, 1939).

Demarest, Mark, "The Fluidity of Identity: Frater VIII, Harry J. Gardener and Harry Lawrence Juhnke," *Chasing Down Emma*, https://ehbritten.blogspot.com/2016/03/the-fluidity-of-identity-frater-vii.html (posted March 3, 2016, accessed February 12, 2022).

de Prati, Gioacchino, "Letters on Tellurism, Commonly Called Animal Magnetism," *The Shepherd*, 1834-1835; repr. *Trilithon* 1 (2014), pp. 76–106.

Deslippe, Philip, "From Maharaj to Maham Tantric: the construction of Yogi Bhajan's Kundalini Yoga," *Sikh Formations* vol. 6 no. 3 (December 2012), pp. 369–387.

Dumont, Theron Q., *The Solar Plexus or Abdominal Brain* (Chicago, IL: Advanced Thought, 1920).

Fortune, Dion, *The Esoteric Philosophy of Love and Marriage* and *The Problem of Purity* (Wellingborough, UK: Aquarian, 1988).

Gardener, Harry J., *Five Fold Life Extension Course* (Los Angeles, CA: Harry J. Gardener, 1957).

Gardener, Harry J., *The Golden Gate to the Garden of Allah* (Los Angeles, CA: The Golden Dawn Press, 1944).

Gardener, Harry J., *Money, Magic, and Mystery In My Life* (Los Angeles, CA: Harry J. Gardener, 1957).

Gardener, Harry J., *Outwitting Tomorrow* (Los Angeles, CA: The Golden Dawn Press, 1934).

Gardener, Harry J., *Streamline Minds* (Los Angeles, CA: Harry J. Gardenerr, 1936).

Gardener, Harry J., *The Rose-Cross Clan* (Los Angeles, CA: The Golden Dawn Press, 1949).

Gardener, Harry J., *The Secret Science of Life* (Los Angeles, CA: Harry J. Gardener, 1942).

Gardener, Harry J., *Turn Back The Years* (Los Angeles, CA: Harry J. Gardener, 1942).

Gardener, Harry J., *What's Next 1961* (Los Angeles, CA: Harry J. Gardener, 1961).

Goldberg, Elliott, *The Path of Modern Yoga* (Rochester, VT: Inner Traditions, 2016).

Hall, Manly P., *Man, Grand Symbol of the Mysteries* (Los Angeles, CA: Philosophical Research Society, 1972).

Hall, Manly P., *Koyasan: Sanctuary of Esoteric Buddhism* (Los Angeles, CA: Philosophical Research Society, 1970).

Hall, Manly P., *Meditation Symbols in Eastern & Western Mysticism* (rev. ed.., Los Angeles; Philosophical Research Society, 1988).

Hall, Manly P., *The Occult Anatomy of Man* (Los Angeles, CA: Philosophical Research Society, 1937).

Hall, Manly P., *Talks to Students on Occult Philosophy* (rev. ed., Los Angeles, CA: Philosophical Research Society, 1975).

Hall, Manly P., *The Secret Teachings of All Ages* (rev. ed., Los Angeles, CA: Philosophical Research Society, 1988).

Hay, William Howard, *Health Via Food* (East Aurora, NY: Sun-Diet Health Service, 1929).

Heindel, Augusta Foss, *Astrology and the Ductless Glands* (Oceanside, CA: Rosicrucian Fellowship, 1936).

Heindel, Max, *The Message of the Stars* (Oceanside, CA: Rosicrucian Fellowship, 1927).

Heindel, Max, *The Rosicrucian Cosmo-Conception* (Seattle, WA: Rosicrucian Fellowship, 1909).

Heindel, Max, *The Vital Body* (Oceanside, CA: Rosicrucian Fellowship, 1950).

Judge, William Quan, *The Yoga Aphorisms of Patanjali* (New York, NY: The Path, 1889).

Judson, Abby A., *Development of Mediumship by Terrestrial Magnetism* (Minneapolis, MN: Alfred Roper, 1891).

Kieser, Dietrich Georg von, *System des Tellurismus oder thierischen Magnetismus* (Leipzig: F.L. Herbig, 1826).

Kneipp, Sebastian, *The Kneipp Cure*, trans. Henry F. Charles (New York, NY: Kneipp Cure Publishing, 1896).

Kraig, Donald Michael, *Modern Magick* (St. Paul, MN: Llewellyn, 1985).

Krishna, Gopi, *Kundalini: The Evolutionary Energy in Man* (Boulder, CO: Shambhala, 1971).

McClenon, James, *Deviant Science* (Philadelphia, PA: University of Pennsylvania Press, 1984).

Motoyama, Hiroshi, *Theories of the Chakras* (Wheaton, IL: Theosophical Press, 1981).

Plummer, George Winslow, *Rosicrucian Fundamentals* (New York, NY: Flame Press, 1920).

Plummer, George Winslow, *Rosicrucian Manual* (New York, NY: Mercury, 1923).

Plummer, George Winslow, *Rosicrucian Symbology* (New York, NY: Macoy, 1916).

Plummer, George Winslow, *Societas Rosicruciana in America Correspondence Lessons, Spiritual Alchemy Series* (New York, NY: privately printed, n.d.).

Plummer, George Winslow, "Those Alchemists—Our Glands," undated lecture (https://sria.org/those-alchemists-our-glands/,accessed 8/21/2021).

Powell, A.E., *The Etheric Double* (London: Theosophical Society, 1925).

Pratidinhi, Bhavanarao Pant, *The Ten-Point Way to Health* (London: J.M. Dent & Sons, 1938).

Ramacharaka, Yogi (William Walker Atkinson), *Hatha Yoga, or the Yogi Philosophy of Physical Well-Being* (Chicago, IL: Yogi Publication Society, 1905).

Ramacharaka, Yogi (William Walker Atkinson), *The Hindu-Yogi System of Practical Water Cure* (Chicago, IL: Yogi Publication Society, 1908).

Raux, Emile (Charles B. Roth), *Hindu Secrets of Virility and Rejuvenation* (Denver, CO: Basic Science Fellowship, 1939).

Regardie, Israel, *The Golden Dawn* (7th rev. ed., Woodbury, MN: Llewellyn, 2015).

Regardie, Israel, *The Middle Pillar* (Chicago, IL: Aries Press, 1938).

Reichenbach, Karl von, *Researches on Magnetism, Electricity, Heat, Light, Crystallization, and Chemical Attraction, in their Relation to the Vital Force*, trans. William Gregory (London: Taylor, Walton, and Maberly, 1850).

Rele, Vasant G., *The Mysterious Kundalini* (Bombay: D.P. Taraporevala Sons, 1931).

Roth, Charles B. *See* Raux, Emil

Sahagun, Louis, *Master of the Mysteries: The Life of Manly Palmer Hall* (Port Townsend, WA: Process Media, 2008).

Seton, Julia, *The Psychology of the Solar Plexus and Subconscious Mind* (New York, NY: Edward J. Clode, 1914).

Sivananda, Sri Swami, *Kundalini Yoga* (Shivanandanagar, India: Divine Life Society, 1980).

Smedley, Caroline Anne, *Ladies' Manual of Practical Hydropathy, Not the Cold Water System* (London: James Blackwood & Co., 1878).

Smythe, F.M.J., *Fire, Air, Earth, and Water* (Los Angeles, CA: Mid-Day Press, 1944).

Steiner, Rudolf, *The Way of Initiation, or How to Attain Knowledge of Higher Worlds* (London: Theosophical Society, 1908).

Towne, Elizabeth, *Just How to Wake the Solar Plexus* (Holyoke, MA: By the author, 1907).

Trall, R.T., *Hydropathic Encyclopedia*, 2 vols. (New York, NY: Fowlers & Wells, 1854).

Virginia, Karena, and Dharm Khalsa, *Essential Kundalini Yoga* (Boulder, CO: Sounds True, 2017).

Watt, Jerry, "Influence of Others in the Original Five Tibetans Book, *The Eye of Revelation*." https://t5t.com/the-influence-of-others-on-the-five-tibetans, accessed February 16, 2022.

Weintraub, Skye, *Natural Healing with Cell Salts* (Pleasant Grove, UT: Woodland, 1996).

Witt, Carolinda, *The 5 Tibetans* (Avalon, NSW, Australia: UnMind, 2008).

Online Archives

Nearly all the source material used in the research project that resulted in this book is long out of copyright and can be found online in PDF format. The two most important archives I used in my research, as mentioned in the introduction, are Archive.org (https://archive.org) and IAPSOP, the International Association for the Preservation of Spiritualist and Occult Periodicals (https://iapsop.org). For those interested in following up some of the clues mentioned in the first chapter, the latter archive has a large collection of the writings of Harry J. Gardener in its collection of occult lessons and correspondence courses at https://iapsop.org/ssoc/.

INDEX

Printed in the USA
CPSIA information can be obtained
at www.ICGtesting.com
JSHW011728201023
50587JS00003B/6